Current Challenges and Advances in Organ Donation and Transplantation

Edited by Georgios Tsoulfas

Published in London, United Kingdom

Current Challenges and Advances in Organ Donation and Transplantation
http://dx.doi.org/10.5772/intechopen.102229
Edited by Georgios Tsoulfas

Contributors
Nadeem Ahmad Khan, Taqi Taufique Khan, Akshay Kumar, Sania Thite, Varad Wazarkar, Kamal Ayyat, Jesus Gomez Abraham, Suresh Keshavamurthy, Sahar Khoshravesh, Dilar Costa, Joana Silva, Stella Vasileiadou, Nikolaos Antoniadis, Georgios Katsanos, Georgios Tsoulfas, Athanasios Kofinas, Konstantina-Eleni Karakasi, Wenshi Jiang, Xiaotong Wu, Liansheng Ma, Jing Shu, Juan Yan, Yajie Ma, Xiangxiang He, Liming Yang, Karen R.V. Francis-Cummings, Kudirat Busari, Abigail Garba

First published in London, United Kingdom, 2023 by IntechOpen
IntechOpen is the global imprint of INTECHOPEN LIMITED, registered in England and Wales, registration number: 11086078, 5 Princes Gate Court, London, SW7 2QJ, United Kingdom

British Library Cataloguing-in-Publication Data
A catalogue record for this book is available from the British Library

Additional hard and PDF copies can be obtained from orders@intechopen.com

Current Challenges and Advances in Organ Donation and Transplantation
Edited by Georgios Tsoulfas
p. cm.
Print ISBN 978-1-83768-005-4
Online ISBN 978-1-83768-006-1
eBook (PDF) ISBN 978-1-83768-007-8

Meet the editor

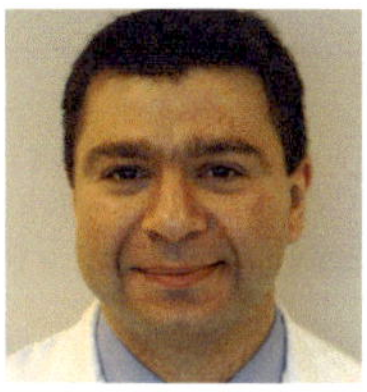

Dr. Georgios Tsoulfas received his medical degree from Brown University School of Medicine, USA, and completed his general surgery residency at the University of Iowa Hospitals and Clinics, USA, as well as a transplant research fellowship at the Starzl Transplant Institute at the University of Pittsburgh, USA. He then completed a two-year transplantation surgery fellowship at Massachusetts General Hospital, Harvard Medical School, USA, and then joined the Division of Solid Organ Transplantation and Hepatobiliary Surgery, University of Rochester Medical Center, USA, as Assistant Professor of Surgery. He is currently living in Greece, where he is a Professor of Transplantation Surgery and chief of the Department of Transplantation Surgery, at Aristotle University School of Medicine. He has published more than 180 papers in peer-reviewed journals and 30 book chapters. He is a reviewer for more than forty international journals and an editorial board member of several others. Dr. Tsoulfas has served as chair of the International Relations Committee of the American College of Surgeons and world president of the International College of Surgeons.

Contents

Preface **IX**

Section 1
Organization of Organ Donation **1**

Chapter 1 **3**
Therapeutic Regimen Adherence and Risk of Renal Graft Loss: Nurse Interventions
by Dilar Costa and Joana Silva

Chapter 2 **19**
Empower the Science of Organ Donation by Multidisciplinary Collaboration
by Wenshi Jiang, Xiaotong Wu, Liansheng Ma, Jing Shu, Juan Yan, Liming Yang, Yajie Ma and Xiangxiang He

Section 2
Ethical and Religious Issues in Organ Donation **35**

Chapter 3 **37**
Altruistic Kidney Donation: Overview and Ethical Considerations
by Kudirat Busari and Abigail Garba

Chapter 4 **49**
Organ Donation: Demand and Supply
by Nadeem Ahmad Khan and Taqi Taufique Khan

Chapter 5 **59**
Nauseous Nexus between the Organ Industry and the Risks of Illegal Organ Harvesting
by Karen R.V. Francis-Cummings

Chapter 6 **73**
Organ Donation in Islam
by Sahar Khoshravesh

Section 3
Advances in Organ Donation 85

Chapter 7 87
Recent Advances and Outcomes in Heart and Lung Transplantation
by Akshay Kumar, Sania Thite, Varad Wazarkar, Kamal Ayyat, Jesus Gomez Abraham and Suresh Keshavamurthy

Chapter 8 115
Machine Perfusion Strategies in Liver and Renal Transplantation
by Stella Vasileiadou, Nikolaos Antoniadis, Athanasios Kofinas, Konstantina-Eleni Karakasi, Georgios Katsanos and Georgios Tsoulfas

Preface

One of the most interesting and challenging fields of medicine and surgery is organ donation and transplantation. It is a field that has made tremendous strides during the last few decades through the combined input and efforts of scientists from various specialties including surgeons, hepatologists, nephrologists, immunologists, ethicists, and infectious disease specialists. What started as a dream of pioneers in the field has become a reality for the thousands of patients whose lives can now be saved and improved. However, challenges remain significant, as do the expectations, for what was once an experimental treatment could eventually become the future of medicine because it involves most organs including the heart, lungs, eyes, liver, kidneys, pancreas, and small intestine.

Written by an excellent group of world authorities, this book presents the challenges in the field of organ donation and transplantation, including ethical, legal, and medical issues, as well as the technical and immunological problems facing experts involved in the care of transplant patients. In addition to the knowledge shared, the authors provide their personal clinical experience, making this book an extremely useful tool for every scientist and physician practicing in the field of transplantation.

The book is divided into three sections on organ donation and transplantation. The chapters include information on the current state and different types of donation, the challenges identified in increasing donations as well as potential solutions.

This book is a worthy contribution to the literature on organ donation and transplantation. It is designed for scientists, physicians, and surgeons across various specialties who are invested in improving the lives of transplant patients.

Georgios Tsoulfas, MD, Ph.D., FICS, FACS
Professor of Transplantation Surgery,
Chief Department of Transplantation Surgery,
Aristotle University of Thessaloniki School of Medicine,
Thessaloniki, Greece

Section 1

Organization of Organ Donation

Chapter 1

Therapeutic Regimen Adherence and Risk of Renal Graft Loss: Nurse Interventions

Dilar Costa and Joana Silva

Abstract

Kidney transplantation is considered the best therapeutic option and survival is dependent on adherence to the drug regimen. Adherence to the therapeutic regime thus becomes the key to success. However, the literature shows that not all patients are adherent, and readmission due to graft dysfunction is a reality. Although a direct relationship between adherence to the therapeutic regimen and graft dysfunction cannot be attributed, the issue of adherence is far from not deserving the attention of health professionals. This text aims to identify the importance of nursing interventions in promoting adherence to the therapeutic regimen. In an exploratory approach to the process of adherence, and reflecting on concordance and its relevance to adherence, given the heterogeneity of both definitions, we aimed to study the nurses' role and the type of interventions to promote adherence to the therapeutic regimen in transplanted renal patients. We conclude that education and counselling are the predominant interventions and that concordance is part of this practice, where the expected outcome is kidney graft survival as a consequence of adherence to the therapeutic regimen.

Keywords: adherence to the therapeutic regimen, patient compliance, adherence, concordance, nurse interventions, nurse care, renal allograft, renal transplantation, renal recipients

1. Introduction

Kidney transplantation is recognised in the medical literature as the best therapeutic option in end-stage chronic kidney disease [1, 2].

There are both clinical and non-clinical reasons to believe that kidney transplantation is beneficial for the person with end-stage renal disease because it reduces cardiovascular risk from 9.0 to 3.5–5.0% per year for patients who remain on dialysis. Added to this are the numerous benefits associated with better quality of life, more freedom (not being dependent on dialysis), more time for daily activities (time gained from not being dependent on dialysis), reduced symptoms such as fatigue, sleep disturbances and, as hypothesised, more work activity [3, 4].

Adherence to the therapeutic regimen of transplanted kidney patients is fundamental in preventing kidney graft rejection, complications, and re-hospitalisations with increased costs for the person and the health system [5].

There is much evidence of the importance of adherence to the therapeutic regimen for kidney transplant patients, highlighting the consequences of non-adherence and giving depth to the benefits that adherence evokes, linking it to processes of well-being and good health.

The direct relationship between adherence and satisfactory health outcomes is perceived, and there are numerous references that report changing behaviours, modifying diet, managing medication, changing routines, and adopting healthy lifestyles, as a bridge to a long life with the kidney graft and better quality of life [6–8].

An indispensable component of kidney graft survival is adherence to the therapeutic regimen, which, although it extends beyond medication adherence to include dietary compliance and lifestyle changes, has mainly been studied on the pharmacological side [9–12].

In one study the authors state that the probability of losing the kidney graft is seven times higher in the group of people not adherent to immunosuppressive medication, a reason in itself sufficient to capture the attention of the scientific community [3].

Some studies have tried to provide an empirical response to this problem, focusing on other aspects that are part of the therapeutic regimen. The results of the study by Gheih and colleagues reveal a clear preference of participants for the adherence to immunosuppressive medication (97.0%), but also show high values of adherence to low-fat diet (73.0%), infection prevention (89.0%), mouth care (brushing of teeth after meals) (37.0%), and physical exercise (walking) (23.0%). Lower adherence values were found in the activities related to monitoring water intake (12.0%), blood pressure (10.0%), temperature (6.0%), and urine output monitoring (2.0%) [7].

Adhikari and colleagues consider that lifestyle modifications have a high weighting in the success of kidney transplantation, however, the levels of adherence achieved by participants for all lifestyle dimensions assessed were low (64.1%), although with strong expression in some dimensions, particularly with regard to self-monitoring (89.54%), medical appointments (88.23%), infection prevention (93.46%), and dietary compliance (83.66%) [8].

These results seem to be in line with what we have previously said about the possible relationship between kidney graft survival and adherence to the therapeutic regimen in its broadest sense.

In this field of intervention, the multiplicity of factors associated with therapeutic adherence moves different actors and approaches. Innovative and pioneering, some projects evoke the individual and collective dimension of action [13–16].

It is interesting to mention that the individual action of a health professional does not potentiate change, but the articulation between health professionals. Change occurs thanks to the action of the individual and groups, such as health professionals, family, network of friends, amongst others.

From time to time there are also great leaps due to social, economic, and political transformations, but it is necessary to invest at a personal level (of the individual and their families) since individual and collective investments are dimensions that coexist, interact, and complement each other, being essential for the success of adherence to the therapeutic regime.

Thus, we have a clear perception of the need for interdependence between all participants in the process. The awareness of the existence of multiple actors and interdependencies in changing behaviours and lifestyles and the respect for each one's field of intervention is a common emphasis amongst nurses.

This professional group often assumes the pivotal position by managing the therapeutic plan with the patient and his/her family, which often involves the orientations of different professionals. All are the reason for success or failure, in a process whose dynamics is made of this interaction [17].

But the most important result with regard to practices promoting adherence to the therapeutic regimen is the empowerment of the patient and compliance with that regimen.

Adherence to the therapeutic regimen involves transitions and adaptations, which brings us to a great challenge if we consider that the trends verified in the literature consecrate a low adherence or non-adherence to the therapeutic regimen.

According to the World Health Organisation (WHO) about 50.0% of chronically ill patients do not adhere to the therapeutic regimen [18].

The literature gives us a clear idea of the prevalence of non-adherence amongst kidney transplant recipients (28.0%) and the implications of non-adherence to immunosuppressive therapy on health outcomes, episodes of graft rejection (20.0%) and organ loss (16.0%) [19].

A second point to be considered is the method used to measure adherence to therapy. The values vary between 2.0 and 67.0%, and the causes of conditioning adherence to the announced values are strongly linked to the operationalisation of the definitions and the measurement methods used. The indicators of adherence used vary between "taking compliance", "dosing compliance", "timing compliance", amongst others.

The methods used include electronic monitoring, which also differ, such as the Medication Event Monitoring System (MEMS), the Short Message Service (SMS) and, more recently, technology based on digestible Integrated Circuits (ICs). Additionally, traditional methods such as patient reports and diaries, direct observation of therapy administration, pill counting, measurement of the concentration of the drug or its metabolite in the blood, and measurement of a biomarker in the blood are also used [20–23].

These two aspects of therapeutic adherence, although distinct, are strongly interconnected. In fact, the traditional method and the more recent methods that employ technology play a primordial role in the context of promoting therapeutic adherence in individuals. Conversely, we could say that the variety of methods does not give us a single standard, the desired gold standard, central to a consensual explanation of therapeutic adherence by the scientific community.

Although international statistics are not very favourable in this area, the therapeutic alliance between the kidney transplant patient and the nurse, marked by their proximity, may intensify the relationship, translating into a greater capacity of the patient to manage his/her therapeutic regimen and annul the interferences and obstacles that contribute to non-adherence.

But what is meant by medication adherence and therapeutic adherence?

The concept has evolved over time, but there is no consensus amongst authors on its definition. The literature offers us different perspectives of therapeutic adherence, as we will see below.

2. Definition of adherence therapeutic

As previously stated, the definition of adherence to the therapeutic regimen is not consensual amongst authors and has evolved over time [24].

It has captured the interest of the scientific community, but although numerous studies from different disciplines have been developed to explain the phenomenon, it is still a worldwide problem.

For the nursing discipline, and based on the International Council of Nurses (ICN) definition, adherence to the therapeutic regimen is defined as adherence behaviour in a broader perspective, namely: "self-initiated action to promote well-being; recovery and rehabilitation; following guidelines without deviations; engaged in a set of actions or behaviours. Complies with treatment regimen; takes medicines as prescribed; changes behaviour for the better, signs of healing, seeks medicines on indicated date, internalises the value of a health behaviour, and obeys instructions regarding treatment. (Often associated with support from family and people who are important to the client, knowledge about medicines and disease process, client motivation, relationship between health professional and client)" ([25], p. 2).

However, the concept itself is somewhat paradoxical. If adherence is the expected outcome, it should prefigure a patient-centred approach, since one can hardly separate people from their circumstances. This means that the patient will have to be an actor and not just a spectator, to be a subject and not an object, to intervene and not just assist, in other words, the patient should not lose his autonomy in the treatment process. Thus, the importance of the patient's action in his/her therapeutic process is equated. The perspective is dialectical between the actors and the various levels of contexts. The concept of adherence has demonstrated shortcomings by denying the patient this possibility. The awareness of the importance of the alliance and negotiation between health professionals and patients in managing the therapeutic regimen gives relevance to the concept of concordance, which aggregates all these attributes.

It is interesting to note that the concept of concordance is harmonised with the new paradigm of care provision, person-centred models, which see the individual as participants in their therapeutic process, according to their preferences, values, and expectations. Concordance implies working in partnership with the person [26].

Trust and negotiation are the foundations for building this partnership, where everyone feels involved, concentrating efforts towards a common goal that is possible to achieve due to the work that each one performs within the partnership. In other words, a relationship between equals with shared objectives, as opposed to a paternalistic approach [27].

A second point to be considered is the nurse-patient relationship, taking into account its importance in obtaining and sustaining agreement. The communication established based on trust, articulated with understanding, tolerance, and respect for the patient's needs, makes that within this framework the care is negotiated and meets the common interests, in a situation of perfect balance [28].

Within the framework of concordance, the understanding between the parties involved in the therapeutic process about the responsibilities from the perspective of assigning the roles that each one will have to assume stands out. The aim is to eliminate the patient's passivity and empower them to make informed decisions.

Imogene King's theory of Goal attainment (1981) highlights, based on its process of interaction-transaction, the nurse's role in helping patients achieve their goals. A key feature of this process is the participation of the nurse and the patient in defining the goals and exploring the resources to achieve them. This is in line with the principles and philosophy of the nursing profession itself, i.e., empowering the patient for self-care [29].

Returning to the issue of therapeutic regime management one can glimpse that skills and competencies are needed to manage the therapeutic regime and that often these skills have to be learned, being in fact a self-care activity. In a situation of interaction between nurse and patient, it is up to both to assess the patient's ability to manage his/her therapeutic regimen. Concordance establishes the therapeutic alliance between the patient and the nurse, a relationship of equals, however, the patient is recognised as the expert of his/her own life. Defending this vision, the World Health Organisation (WHO), in the Ottawa Convention (1986), ratified the fundamental right of all people to be part of their own health care. From then on, the patient's autonomy came to occupy a prominent place in nursing care [30].

For both, there are no longer margins or spaces where asymmetric power relations could emerge. In the last 30 years, the relationship between patients and health professionals has undergone important changes, with the patient assuming greater control in his/her health decisions. This relationship is also closely associated with the disease model that dominates each era [31].

The new model of care, centred on the patient and based on a holistic perspective, seeks to explore the patient's perspectives and expectations, and understand them in their particular context. It implies sharing responsibility, involving the patient in decisions, and making him/her responsible for his/her health [32]. This model assumes great importance, especially at a time marked by the upsurge of chronic and lifestyle-related diseases [33].

We thus asked ourselves about the place of concordance in the practice of care in the promotion of behaviours of adherence to the therapeutic regime. Does the model have the effervescence and synergy that have permeated practices in recent decades? (I am only quoting the paternalistic model that still prevails in our health institutions) How have care practices been configured in the new model of care provision?

Authors such as Snowden [26], Gardner [34], point out that concordance is in simultaneity with the principles and values of the nursing profession when they "make the care of people your first concern, treating them as individuals and respecting their dignity" ([35], p. 2).

As a response to a care context marked by the holistic model as opposed to the previous approach, which proved to be an inefficient model, today we witness an interest in the centrality of the patient in the disease process and in meeting their needs. For Beresford [36], in order to optimise concordance, holism should be the goal of care provision and communication should be the heart of patient-centred care [37].

This new model of care is, however, a challenge in clinical settings, as patients move to other settings, whether to other healthcare institutions or to home. This increases the difficulty in negotiating the goals and the means to achieve them.

However, it is important to situate this positions between professionals and patients in a context of growing uncertainty which, from the point of view of care production, are increasing, such as new economic issues and new publics, in which in the same sociological profile of the public different ways of seeing may be inscribed.

However, it is public knowledge that health outcomes improve when patients are involved in their therapeutic process, working together with health professionals, as resources are used more effectively and efficiently. On the other hand, professionals feel more satisfied because their work has contributed to improving those outcomes. For the Health Department, the articulation of these two aspects shows that patients and health professionals are stakeholders in the success of concordance throughout nursing practice [38].

In line with a profession that values the uniqueness of the patient, which favours active listening, and advocates on behalf of the patient, we sought to analyse which nursing interventions are implemented by nurses to promote therapeutic adherence.

According to Giddens' sociology, true shared decision-making results from the sharing of power. For the author, power is defined as the ability to "make it happen", to "produce effects" in the societal world. If power is the ability to influence a course of events, in this particular case of the transition of the recently transplanted patient from hospital to home, resources are any strategies that increase this ability of the patient, that is, that provide the patient with the necessary tools to manage his therapeutic regimen [39].

Interestingly, despite advocating a patient-centred care model, in the concordance equation, the patients' non-participation in their therapeutic process is in the numerator, i.e., the part of the number in which concordance is used by health professionals, in this case, nurses. According to the literature, one of the common complaints of patients is that their opinions, needs, and expectations are not considered in decisions about their health [40].

It thus seems plausible to argue that concordance-based care exponentially increases the chance of adherence, whilst the opposite may eventually contribute to non-adherence to the therapeutic regime.

There is a plethora of studies addressing this issue, showing the magnitude of its intensity on the patient and the health system.

Non-adherence behaviours lead to inadequate control of the disease, putting the patient at great risk due to the emergence of adverse effects.

Dew and colleagues studied the non-adherence rates of all types of organ transplantation, and, strangely, despite the high number of non-adherent transplant recipients across the various dimensions of the therapeutic regimen, the number of kidney transplant representative's non-adherent to immunosuppressive medication rises relative to other recipients (36 cases per 100 patients per Year vs. 7 to 15 cases) [41].

Life expectancy also decreases four times more in the group of non-adherent transplant recipients [42]. We are thus elucidated about one of the striking features of the international reality in the field of adherence to the therapeutic regime, without exception. Added to this is the problem of growing discontinuity between healthcare services (although in recent years there are signs that this trend is being reversed, with a gradual increase in the articulation between healthcare institutions and patient follow-up).

Chronic illness, because it persists over time, requires continuous monitoring by health professionals in order to promote adherence to the therapeutic regime [43].

Two distinct but overlapping notions lead us to the concept of self-management and self-care. Indeed, we found that the term self-management is associated with the term self-care and, precisely in chronic diseases, aims to help patients maintain their well-being. It should be noted that chronic disease follows a trajectory marked by transitions and adaptations that involves a set of activities, such as medication management, adherence to a specific diet, changes in behaviours and lifestyles, which requires the action of the patient and the health professional to ensure an active life and a higher quality of life [44].

This would reinforce the proximity of adherence to the notions of self-management and self-care. We draw attention to the fact that both terms have the same purpose as adherence: to establish care partnerships and enable or empower the patient to take action.

Considering the transition as a medical and nursing phenomenon, nurses should analyse the present and predictable effects of the transition to transplantation. Transplant recipients have many tasks to perform: taking medication (according to medical prescription), changes in lifestyle, including diet, physical exercise, monitoring of signs and symptoms of organ rejection, monitoring of complications (infections), monitoring of fluid intake and elimination, monitoring of blood pressure and blood glucose, performance of complementary diagnostic tests, visits to consultations, smoking cessation, management of stress and emotions, and performance of other self-care activities essential to a good health status [6–8].

Briefly, after kidney transplantation, adaptation to the new condition creates the need for organ recipients, now in a newly acquired situation, to integrate the recommendations of the therapeutic regimen regarding immunosuppressive medication, lifestyles, routines, social roles, and emotional challenges [45].

Indeed, adherence becomes the major reason to ensure the survival of the kidney graft without the trade-off of losing the organ due to inadequate self-care. If patients can understand the importance of therapeutic compliance, they can also begin to understand its implications on their lives at various levels [46].

We cannot but agree with the statement of these authors regarding the relevance of adherence to the therapeutic regimen as a means to counteract the harmful consequences of non-adherence and to recognise the nurse's intervention as vital, as it may contribute to the perception of the change that begins in the transition to the new condition, that is, when the person is admitted for transplantation.

In fact, according to their role in the health team, nurses play a central role in the management of the therapeutic regime, identifying difficulties and constraints, integrating the different aspects of the therapeutic regime, and constituting themselves as partners and resources [17].

According to the WHO, nurses are in a privileged position to diagnose, intervene, and assess results in aspects related to therapeutic adherence [18].

Evidently, the role of nurses is a key element in the framework of therapeutic adherence [47, 48], which calls for educational and behavioural strategies to promote adherence.

In addition to nurses, the presence of other health professionals, family, communities, and society are fundamental to promote adherence. Thus, a field of proposals is created in which the transplanted person will learn to manage his therapeutic regimen according to his needs [36].

Following the above, our objective is to identify the nursing interventions that promote therapeutic adherence amongst kidney transplant recipients, which leads us to the following research question: What are the nursing interventions that promote therapeutic adherence amongst kidney transplant recipients?

In the following section, we aim to answer this question.

3. Nursing interventions to promote adherence therapeutic

Therapeutic adherence is a current issue and is part of the "habitus" of nursing professionals' actions, with terms such as "information", "education", "partnership", "self-care", and "empowerment" as frames of reference; in short, the essential components for therapeutic self-management.

Aiming to identify in the literature the nursing interventions promoting adherence to the therapeutic regimen, we used Bleser and colleagues' classification for this purpose [49]:

1. Educational/cognitive interventions that communicate information related to kidney transplantation, by telephone, email, face-to-face, in written or verbal form.

2. Counselling/behavioural interventions, which aim to direct, adapt, and promote appropriate adherence behaviours.

3. Psycho-affective interventions, which include social support from significant others and health professionals.

We also determined the level of intervention according to the ecological model of McLeroy and colleagues [50]. For the authors, interventions can be classified into four levels, namely:

1. Patient level Interventions, directed only to the sick person, which include the above-mentioned categories of intervention (educational/cognitive, counselling/behaviour, and psychologic/affective Interventions).

2. Interventions at the micro level or interpersonal level, which refer to strategies focused on the patient/health care professional interaction, such as the perception of the quality of the relationship between them and the communication style practiced.

3. Interventions at the meso level, which are related to the characteristics of the health care organisation where care occurs, hospital or other health care institution, for example, how continuity of care is ensured or the articulation of skills amongst professionals.

4. Interventions at the macro level, which refer to interventions focused on the health system or the community where the patient lives, for example, health insurance, the patient's expenditure on medication and, finally, the combination of the different levels reported interventions integrating more than one of the levels described.

Studies were found in the literature showing education as a resource to empower the patient and enable him/her to self-manage the therapeutic regime.

Several theories and theoretical models are at the basis of these educational programs. And, although adherence to the therapeutic regimen is a multidisciplinary work, in this case we only portray the nurse's role in this process.

Table 1 shows the interventions developed by nursing professionals to promote adherence to the therapeutic regimen.

The data analysed show us that there are two types of interventions to improve therapeutic adherence: educational and behavioural interventions.

Education is the privileged intervention in most studies, but the way it is administered, and the contents taught show some different contours between the studies.

Information and communication technologies are essential tools for education and training, imposing greater autonomy to the patient.

This generates the need for nursing professionals to develop flexible education programs in which the internet and multimedia resources gain relevance. Video is one of the resources widely used by nursing professionals [51].

Educational interventions promote the knowledge of the person and/or caregiver about the disease and treatment, using a diversity of tools, whether paper-based, audiovisual, social media, or discussion.

On the other hand, behavioural interventions aim to help the person gain skills and/or competencies through training, counselling to manage their therapeutic regime.

Rocha and colleagues formulate an educational plan that was based on the learning styles of each participant. The methods used varied between subjects, and the

Interventions	Dimensions			Level
	Cognitive-INFORMATIONAL	Behaviour	Affective	
Educational plan specific to each identified learning style (visual, aural, read/write, kinesthetic) and educational sessions [51].	Informative sessions Video presentation Orientation manual	Nurse couselling		Patient-individual
Transplant-TAVIE 3 interactive Web-based sessions. Virtual nurse based on Social Learning Theory and Behaviour Changes Techniques [52]	Teaching, feedback Role models (experiences of others' patients)	Positive Reinforcement	Social interaction	Patient-individual
SystemCHANGE Interventions used the Deming's Plan-Do-Check-Act to redesign personal environment system and daily health behaviour routines. Educational Intervention. Using healthy living transplant brochures-Control Group In-person visit Telephone calls	Education SystemCHANGE teaches patients to use person-level. Quality improvement strategies to link adherence to established daily routines, environmental cues, and supportive people. Attention Control (Patient Education) Transplant Health-Related Brochures. Report	In-person visit Small experiments of medical adherence solutions.	Nurse Orientation Telephone calls to receive feedback (report) and discuss. Telephone call to review transplant-related education materials. Support of significant others. Assess individual system and environment (SystemCHANGE). Assess MA (EM) Feedback	Patient (individual) micro (immediate environmental setting of family, peers, health services, workplace). Meso (interrelations between family, health care provider, employer)
The Disease Guidance Manual delivered on admission. Health education Nursing intervention based on Health Believe Model. Sign behaviour agreement Daily record Follow-up: • Phone, WeChat/SMS [15].	The Disease Guidance Manual Report	HBM education Feedback	Give encouragement about behaviour change. Interaction: • Telephone call • WeChat • SMS Family support	Patient, micro Meso

Table 1.
Interventions developed by nursing professionals to promote adherence to the therapeutic regímen.

privileged dimensions were cognitive and behavioural. The results showed an increase in medication adherence from the first to third meeting: 16.9% (in the first), 66.1% (in the second), and 79.9% (in the third). The construction of the educational plan was elaborated collaboratively, taking into account the subject's own characteristics, and demonstrated health gains for the patient [51].

The same attitude was taken by Cotê and collegues. In this case, the authors used information technologies, creating an interactive website—Virtual Nurse. The expected results were achieved, namely medication adherence and self-efficacy. Participants found the individualised education interventions to be personalised, easy to understand and self-efficacy promoting. Medication adherence (11.4, range 1–12) and self-efficacy (81.3, range 0–100) scores were high. Perceived health status and quality of life similarly achieved high scores (8.3, in a range of 0–10) [52].

The study by Russell and colleagues implemented an innovative education system, SystemCHANGE, which included home visits and telephone calls. In this system one can observe negotiation as an essential strategy in goal setting and discussion as one of the means to define resources and solutions to identified problems. The results showed differences between the experimental group and the control group in medication adherence at 12 months (large differences in medians, 0.17, 95% CI, 0.06–0.33, $p < .001$). Program implementation lasted six months and follow-up was twelve months [15].

However, achieving adherence to therapy, patient involvement and ensuring the survival of the kidney graft requires knowledge and information. This involves informing, educating, and training the patient and/or caregiver to carry out this task. Precisely education and training are fundamental bases for any society.

We have found that listening to the sick person, respecting them, and having an attitude of trust are the bases for adherence. Telephone contact, email, or face-to-face contact are some strategies that facilitate this process. The active involvement of the person in his treatment is the best strategy for its success [53].

The sequence of such actions is reflected in patient autonomy, the elimination of barriers between health professionals and patients, the relationship between the two parties, and the facilitation of access by all citizens to the resources of the health system, the community and society in general.

Although adherence to the therapeutic regimen is an internationally recognised problem and the ways to solve it have already been studied, there are still problems whose impact is negative for the patient and for society.

4. Conclusion

It can be stated that the issue of adherence to the therapeutic regimen is one of the striking phenomena of kidney transplantation, transversal to all types of organ transplantation, which extends far beyond the simple management of medication, requiring an intervention of all health professionals along the trajectory of the disease in order to empower the patient and/or his family.

Although in recent years there are signs that this trend may be receding in some places, based on a plethora of studies which continue to show the existence of the problem at still high levels of non-adherence, we are generally witnessing the emergence of new models of care which, in themselves, facilitate adherence to the therapeutic regimen.

Within the emerging new models, studies show the importance of the nurses' role in promoting adherence behaviours, which is an inherent characteristic of the profession itself. Nursing care is, by its essence, holistic care, based on communication and therapeutic alliance. Negotiation is a sine qua non condition of this process.

Nurses seek to know the response patterns of the ill person and/or caregiver to the disease or problem that affects them, because only in this way they can help them face that situation. The knowledge of the patients and/or caregivers' needs and difficulties and their potential for autonomy allow for the development of a plan adjusted to these needs. Indeed, all clinical practices are guided by the needs of patients, and kidney transplantation is a real challenge for the patient and his or her family, involving many issues that are fundamental for success. Learning to deal with all these aspects requires knowledge acquisition, skills training, and coaching. The emotional needs connected with all the change must be emphasised, in addition to the stress that uncertainty and change provoke. The aim is to work out a plan with the patient and/or caregiver that allows him/her to make a healthy transition and ensure stability for the new role.

Education and counselling were the most commonly developed interventions by nurses after kidney transplantation. However, since most studies focused on medication adherence and the follow-up period did not exceed 12 months, it is important to develop longitudinal studies to measure the long-term effect of these programmes on kidney transplant survival. On the other hand, the heterogeneity of the instruments used does not ensure that a measurement standard is obtained, nor does it allow knowing the true effect of the interventions developed on adherence to the therapeutic regimen and their long-term impact.

5. Implications for practice

Working on the issue of therapeutic adherence within the new paradigm of health care is essential for the survival of the health system, taking into account the expenditure on health care with chronic diseases resulting from a population living longer and longer. Nurses, due to their characteristics, are equipped with the essential tools to work with patients in the search for the best solutions to their problems/health condition.

Some countries, such as the United Kingdom, are aware that the way forward is to educate, inform, and involve the patient and their family, preparing them to take care of themselves. The nurse, as an agent of change and educator, is in the right place and position to develop this role.

At the end of this reflective journey, we found that the issue of adherence to the therapeutic regimen in kidney transplantation leads to several disruptions, namely the change of perspective in the formulation of the care plan and the long-term follow-up of these patients.

The first rupture related to the care plan is to include the patient in the planning process and offer him/her the information and knowledge he/she needs to make a decision based on the best available evidence. The second rupture is to accompany the patient throughout this process, in favour of the idea of a transition process with an extended temporality. The aim is to ensure a transition whereby individuals emerge endowed with autonomy and are able to obtain the desired result: the success of the transplant.

Conflict of interest

The authors declare no conflict of interest.

Author details

Dilar Costa* and Joana Silva
Centro Hospitalar Universitário Lisboa Norte, Lisbon, Portugal

*Address all correspondence to: dilarcosta@gmail.com

References

[1] Khezerloo S, Mahmoudi H, Sharif Nia H, Vafadar Z. Predictors of self-management among kidney transplant recipients. Urology Journal. 2019;**16**(4):366-371. Available from: https://pubmed.ncbi.nlm.nih.gov/31364096/

[2] Schmid-Mohler G, Schäfer-Keller P, Frei A, Fehr T, Spirig R. A mixed-method study to explore patients' perspective of self-management tasks in the early phase after kidney transplant. Progress in Transplantation. 2014;**24**(1):8-18

[3] Mendonça AEO de, Torres G de V, Salvetti M de G, Alchieri JC, Costa IKF. Mudanças na qualidade de vida após transplante renal e fatores relacionados. Acta Paulista de Enfermagem. 2014;**27**(3):287-292

[4] Pinsky BW, Takemoto SK, Lentine KL, Burroughs TE, Schnitzler MA, Salvalaggio PR. Transplant outcomes and economic costs associated with patient noncompliance to immunosuppression. American Journal of Transplantation. 2009;**9**(11):2597-2606

[5] Hucker A, Bunn F, Carpenter L, Lawrence C, Farrington K, Sharma S. Non-adherence to immunosuppressants following renal transplantation: A protocol for a systematic review. BMJ Open [Internet]. 28 Sep 2017;**7**(9):e015411. Available from: https://www.ncbi.nlm.nih.gov/pmc/articles/PMC5640118/

[6] Nowicka M, Górska M, Nowicka Z, Edyko K, Goździk M, Kurnatowska I. Adherence to pharmacotherapy and lifestyle recommendations among hemodialyzed patients and kidney transplant recipients. Journal of Renal Nutrition. Sep 2021;**31**(5):503-511. DOI: 10.1053/j.jrn.2020.12.006. Epub 21 Feb 26.

[7] Gheith AO, El-Saadany SA, Donia SAA, Salem YM. Compliance with recommended life style behaviors in kidney transplant recipients: Does it matter in living donor kidney transplant? Iranian Journal of Kidney Diseases. 2008;**2**(4):218-226

[8] Adhikari U, Taraphder A, Hazra A, Das T. Compliance of kidney transplant recipients to the recommended lifestyle measures following transplantation. Indian Journal of Transplantation. 2018;**12**(1):17

[9] Kostalova B, Ribaut J, Dobbels F, Gerull S, Mala-Ladova K, Zullig LL, et al. Medication adherence interventions in transplantation lack information on how to implement findings from randomized controlled trials in real-world settings: A systematic review. Transplantation Reviews. 2022;**36**(1):100671

[10] Chen T, Wang Y, Tian D, Zhang J, Xu Q, Lv Q, et al. Follow-up factors contribute to immunosuppressant adherence in kidney transplant recipients. Patient Preference and Adherence. 2022;**16**:2811-2819

[11] Stephenson M, Bradshaw W. Kidney transplantation: Interventions to improve medication adherence. Renal Society of Australasia Journal. 2020;**16**(1):8-12

[12] Cossart AR, Staatz CE, Isbel NM, Campbell SB, Cottrell WN. Exploring transplant medication-taking behaviours in older adult kidney transplant recipients: A qualitative study of semi-structured interviews. Drugs & Aging. 2022;**39**(11):887-898

[13] Zachciał J, Uchmanowicz I, Krajewska M, Banasik M. Adherence to immunosuppressive therapies after kidney transplantation from a biopsychosocial perspective: A cross-sectional study. Journal of Clinical Medicine. 2022;**11**(5):1381

[14] Russell CL, Moore S, Hathaway D, Cheng AL, Chen G, Goggin K. MAGIC Study: Aims, design and methods using SystemCHANGE™ to improve immunosuppressive medication adherence in adult kidney transplant recipients. BMC Nephrology. 16 Jul 2016;**17**(1)

[15] Russell CL, Hathaway D, Remy LM, Aholt D, Clark D, Miller C, et al. Improving medication adherence and outcomes in adult kidney transplant patients using a personal systems approach: SystemCHANGE™ results of the MAGIC randomized clinical trial. American Journal of Transplantation. 2019;**20**(1):125-136

[16] Tang J, Kerklaan J, Wong G, Howell M, Scholes-Robertson N, Guha C, et al. Perspectives of solid organ transplant recipients on medicine-taking: Systematic review of qualitative studies. American Journal of Transplantation. 2021;**21**(10):3369-3387

[17] International Council of Nurses. Catálogo CIPE. Lisboa: Ordem dos Enfermeiros; 2011

[18] Sabaté E. Adherence to Long-Term Therapies:Evidence for Action [Internet]. Geneva: World Health Organization; 2003. Available from: http://www.who.int/chp/knowledge/publications/adherence_full_report.pdf

[19] Denhaerynck K, Dobbels F, Cleemput I, Desmyttere A, Schafer-Keller P, Schaub S, et al. Prevalence, consequences, and determinants of nonadherence in adult renal transplant patients: A literature review. Transplant International. 2005;**18**(10):1121-1133

[20] Shi L, Liu J, Fonseca V, Walker P, Kalsekar A, Pawaskar M. Correlation between adherence rates measured by MEMS and self-reported questionnaires: A meta-analysis. Health and Quality of Life Outcomes. 2010;**8**:99

[21] Garfield S, Clifford S, Eliasson L, Barber N, Willson A. Suitability of measures of self-reported medication adherence for routine clinical use: A systematic review. BMC Medical Research Methodology. Dec 2011;**11**(1). DOI: 10.1186/1471-2288-11-149

[22] Granger BB, Bosworth HB. Medication adherence: Emerging use of technology. Current Opinion in Cardiology [Internet]. 2011;**26**(4):279-287. Available from: https://www.ncbi.nlm.nih.gov/pmc/articles/PMC3756138/

[23] Russo HE, Kirsh WD. Population-based medication adherence programmes: A window of opportunities. World Hospitals and Health Services. 2013;**49**(3):14-17 PMID: 24377142

[24] Cruz RS. Evolução do conceito de adesão à terapêutica. Saúde & Tecnologia [Internet]. 2017;**18**:11-16. Available from: https://journals.ipl.pt/stecnologia/article/view/561

[25] International Council of Nurses. CIPE ®. Versão 2. Classificação Internacional para a Prática de Enfermagem. Lisboa: Ordem dos Enfermeiros; 2015

[26] Snowden A, Marland G. No decision about me without me: Concordance operationalised. Journal of Clinical Nursing. 2012;**22**(9-10):1353-1360

[27] Green J, Jester R. Challenges to concordance: Theories that explain

variations in patient responses. British Journal of Community Nursing. 2019;**24**(10):466-473

[28] McKinnon J. The case for concordance: Value and application in nursing practice. British Journal of Nursing. 2013;**22**(13):766-771

[29] King IM. King's conceptual system, theory of goal attainment, and transaction process in the 21st century. Nursing Science Quarterly. 2007;**20**(2):109-111

[30] Robnik M, Blenkuš DMG, Blenkuš MV, Robnik M, Gabrijelčič M. 30 Years after the Ottawa Charter: Is it Still Relevant in the Face of Future Challenges for Health Promotion? [Internet]. EuroHealthNet Magazine.; 2016. Available from: https://eurohealthnet-magazine.eu/30-years-after-the-ottawa-charter-is-it-still-relevant-in-the-face-of-future-challenges-for-health-promotion/?gclid

[31] Jewson ND. The disappearance of the sick-man from medical cosmology, 1770-1870. International Journal of Epidemiology. 2009;**38**(3):622-633

[32] Ishikawa H, Hashimoto H, Kiuchi T. The evolving concept of "patient-centeredness" in patient–physician communication research. Social Science & Medicine. 2013;**96**:147-153

[33] Global Status Report on Noncommunicable Diseases 2014: Attaining the Nine Global Noncommunicable Diseases Targets; A Shared Responsibility—World | ReliefWeb [Internet]. reliefweb.int.. Available from: https://reliefweb.int/report/world/global-status-report-noncommunicable-diseases-2014-attaining-nine-global?gclid=Cj0KCQiAjbagBhD3ARIsANRrqEv8e0Nr6DULqBVX8E6qMYvuPIK-2ABYKwfQOcgu_mvY0X1mrFVh4dgaAluIEALw_wcB

[34] Gardner CL. Adherence: A concept analysis. International Journal of Nursing Knowledge. 2014;**26**(2):96-101

[35] Nursing & Midwifery Council. The Code: Professional Standards of Practice and Behaviour for Nurses, Midwives and Nursing Associates [Internet]. NMC. Nursing and Midwifery Council; 2018. Available from: https://www.nmc.org.uk/standards/code/

[36] Beresford MJ. Medical reductionism: Lessons from the great philosophers. QJM: An International Journal of Medicine [Internet]. 2010;**103**(9):721-724. Available from: https://academic.oup.com/qjmed/article/103/9/721/1581110

[37] Smith J, Bekker H, Cheater F. Theoretical versus pragmatic design in qualitative research. Nurse Researcher. 2011;**18**(2):39-51

[38] Department of Health. Equity and excellence: Liberating the NHS [Internet]. 2010. Available from: https://assets.publishing.service.gov.uk/government/uploads/system/uploads/attachment_data/file/213823/dh_117794.pdf

[39] Giddens A. Studies in Social and Political Theory (RLE Social Theory). Routledge: Taylor & Francis Group; 2014

[40] Coulter A, Collins A. Making Shared Decision-Making a Reality No Decision about Me, Without Me [Internet]. 2011. Available from: https://www.kingsfund.org.uk/sites/default/files/Making-shared-decision-making-a-reality-paper-Angela-Coulter-Alf-Collins-July-2011_0.pdf

[41] Dew MA, DiMartini AF, De Vito DA, Myaskovsky L, Steel J, Unruh M, et al. Rates and risk factors for nonadherence to the medical regimen after adult solid

organ transplantation. Transplantation. 2007;**83**(7):858-873

[42] Chrisholm-Burns MA, Spivey CA, Wilks SE. Social support and immunosuppressant therapy adherence among adult renal transplant recipients. Clinical Transplantation. 2010;**24**:312-320

[43] Yazdi Zadeh F, Moeini M, Shafie D. Evaluation of the Effect of Adherence to Treatment Regimen Program on Quality of Life in Atrial Fibrillation Patients Hospitalized in Shahid Chamran Hospital in Isfahan in 2017 [Internet]. 2019. Available from: http://saber.ucv.ve/ojs/index.php/rev_lh/article/view/16751

[44] Lorig KR, Holman HR. Self-management education: History, definition, outcomes, and mechanisms. Annals of Behavioral Medicine [Internet]. 2003;**26**(1):1-7. Available from: https://academic.oup.com/abm/article/26/1/1/4630312

[45] Jamieson NJ, Hanson CS, Josephson MA, Gordon EJ, Craig JC, Halleck F, et al. Motivations, challenges, and attitudes to self-management in kidney transplant recipients: A systematic review of qualitative studies. American Journal of Kidney Diseases. 2016;**67**(3):461-478

[46] Been-Dahmen JMJ, Beck DK, Peeters MAC, van der Stege H, Tielen M, van Buren MC, et al. Evaluating the feasibility of a nurse-led self-management support intervention for kidney transplant recipients: A pilot study. BMC Nephrology. 27 Apr 2019;**20**(1):143. DOI: 10.1186/s12882-019-1300-7

[47] Rodriguez G, Utate M, Joseph G, St. Victor T. Oral chemotherapy adherence: A novel nursing intervention using an electronic health record workflow. Clinical Journal of Oncology Nursing. 2017;**21**(2):165-167

[48] Wang J, Yue P, Huang J, Xie X, Ling Y, Jia L, et al. Nursing intervention on the compliance of hemodialysis patients with end-stage renal disease: A meta-analysis. Blood Purification [Internet]. 2017;**45**(1-3):102-109. Available from: https://www.karger.com/Article/FullText/484924

[49] De Bleser L, Matteson M, Dobbels F, Russell C, De Geest S. Interventions to improve medication-adherence after transplantation: A systematic review. Transplant International. 2009;**22**(8):780-797

[50] McLeroy KR, Bibeau D, Steckler A, Glanz K. An ecological perspective on health promotion programs. Health Education Quarterly [Internet]. 1988;**15**(4):351-377. Available from: https://journals.sagepub.com/doi/10.1177/109019818801500401

[51] Rocha DF d, Figueiredo AEPL, Canabarro ST, Sudbrack AW. The importance of educational interventions for adherence to the immunosuppressant treatment program to kidney-transplanted patients. ConScientiae Saúde. 2018;**17**(3):273-280

[52] Côté J, Fortin M-C, Auger P, Rouleau G, Dubois S, Boudreau N, et al. Web-based tailored intervention to support optimal medication adherence among kidney transplant recipients: Pilot parallel-group randomized controlled trial. JMIR Formative Research. 2018;**2**(2):e14

[53] Bugalho A, Carneiro AV. Intervenções para aumentar a adesão terapêutica em patologias crónicas. Lisboa: Centro de Estudos de Medicina Baseada na Evidência; 2004

Chapter 2

Empower the Science of Organ Donation by Multidisciplinary Collaboration

Wenshi Jiang, Xiaotong Wu, Liansheng Ma, Jing Shu, Juan Yan, Liming Yang, Yajie Ma and Xiangxiang He

Abstract

Inter-discipline is formed by the interpenetration and integration of multiple disciplines, which has become a notable trend involving interdisciplinary activities and a combination of research and development. Learned from experience worldwide, the management mode for organ donation and procurement activities varies among countries, but the core of the disciplinary construction of organ donation remains the same. The theoretical basis and practice of organ donation is not purely a matter of coordination, but its ground of knowledge is built upon multidisciplinary integration and its implementation relies on a joint-effort approach and requires collaboration of multiple teams. From the sociological viewpoint, organ donation represents the gift of life for transplant patients, which founds the key element in enhancing the harmony of society. While, from a practical perspective, its professionalism has been widely recognized by the international medical community. As a complex medical and social act, organ donation is a medical-centered subject with sociological, humanistic, ethical, psychologic, and juristic attributes. This chapter will provide an overview of how multidisciplinary collaboration empowers the science of organ donation, followed by the summary of recent efforts taken in China in pursuit of this goal as an example.

Keywords: organ donation, multidisciplinary integration, organ procurement organization, brain death, ICU

1. Introduction

The interdisciplinary approach connects interdependent knowledge and skills from more than one subject area to examine a central theme, which can be adopted to effectively address new problems and challenges facing mankind and represents a general trend in the disciplinary and professional development. In the real world, it is sometimes difficult to further develop knowledge without mutual penetration and supplementation between disciplines. Complex problems have to be solved through the synergy of multiple ideas, methods, tools, and instruments, requiring collaboration and cooperation among multidisciplinary professionals. Quite a few examples including the discovery and application of penicillin show that scientific and technological advances are the outcomes of interdisciplinary cooperation.

To promote interdisciplinary integration, many countries have introduced encouraging policies, launched series of state-level disciplinary research projects, and set up interdisciplinary professional degrees at the college level [1, 2]. Meanwhile, academic activities themed on multidisciplinary integration can be seen more frequently in the recent decade, and more clinical guidelines have been jointly compiled by a multidisciplinary panel of experts to achieve thoughtful solutions to the questions concerned.

Empirical evidence has proven that the knowledge basis of organ donation (OD) is a medical-centered subject with sociological, humanistic, psychological, ethical, and juristic attributes. It represents a typical example of multidisciplinary collaboration driving professional development in the field. In this chapter, we try to explain the necessity and feasibility of adopting multidisciplinary collaboration to advance the OD disciplinary system by analyzing the nature of its bottleneck problems and the key processes, with an introduction of current efforts taken in China to reach such a goal.

2. The necessity of promoting the building of OD discipline system through multidisciplinary collaboration

The professionalism of the OD discipline has been widely recognized by the international academic community, as exemplified by the establishment of the International Society of Organ Donation and Procurement (ISODP) and national/regional professional associations for OD in different countries [3]. This recognition indicates the necessity and feasibility of the building of the OD discipline system as the core to guide daily practice and create academic environment.

The overall goal of building the OD discipline system is to protect the legitimate rights and interests of donors and their families, maximize the transplant benefit of recipients and promote harmonious development of human society through establishing a sound scientific theoretical system with distinct characteristics of social humanity to guide actions and practices. Meanwhile, upon which it also drives, in a sustainable fashion, both the development of professional skills and qualified personnel. The establishment and development of the OD discipline system are in conformity with the goal of "self-sufficiency" in organ donation and organ transplantation (OD and OT).

Empirical evidence shows that the establishment of such a theoretical system and its operation practice requires the collaboration of multidisciplinary expertise and the support of multiple teams. We will explain the details in the paragraphs below and the fact that the OD discipline and OT discipline can develop with their own focus and are mutually reinforcing.

2.1 The solution to bottleneck problems of OD requires the multidisciplinary effort

The sustainable and sound development of OD and OT has been a concern of the international community and local governments, which has been driven by two main factors [4].

Firstly, organ shortage is still a common issue worldwide, despite the fact that the global number of OTs has been increasing in the recent decade. According to data collected by the WHO Global Observatory on Organ Donation and Transplantation, there are more than 1,200,000 patients on a current transplantation waiting list, while only 120,000–130,000 transplants are performed a year globally [5]. In recent years, the outbreak of the COVID-19 pandemic has had a great impact on people's daily life and has posed grave challenges to the building and operating efficiency of OD and OT systems in all countries. In the circumstance that the burden of disease and transplantation demand did not decline, the global OT number in 2020 declined by 17.6% compared with that in 2019 [5].

Secondly, donated organs are valuable national resources, giving OD an attribute of social public welfare [6] and its natural links to society. As advocated in the WHO guiding principles on human cell, tissue, and organ transplantation (WHO guiding principles) [7], OD and OT activities should be strictly regulated by the government of member countries, and illegal organ trading should be prohibited. In order to achieve "self-sufficiency" and sustainability of OT, the development of OD and OT programs needs to be based on legal and ethical requirements, with maintaining equity, transparency, accessibility, high quality, and patients' safety at the core.

By further analyzing the nature of the above requirements, it is not difficult to identify a more in-depth demand: The development of the OD program does not only depend on any single community but also requires the support and participation of multiple parties from various sectors and knowledge transferred from multi-disciplines.

2.2 The whole process of OD requires collaboration among multi-teams

The management mode of organ procurement varies in different countries. Whether built inside medical institutions or being independent outside the hospital, the Organ Procurement Organization (OPO) represents a professional team/organization responsible for the procurement, distribution, and coordination of organ & tissue donation activities at the practical level. The OPO is composed of professionals from different fields such as intensive care medicine, transplantation medicine, anesthesiology, nursing, bioengineering, sociology, psychology, medical ethics and information technology, etc. Its mission and goals are to maximize local donation rate and the number of transplantable organs so as to save more transplant patients and improve their living quality. OPOs and the transplant coordinators serve as a bridge for overall coordination in the entire process at the institutional and individual levels, respectively. Such a collaborative network covers multidisciplinary teams within medical institutions, such as the health care teams in the intensive care unit (ICU), emergency department, neurology department, neurosurgery department, laboratory, transplantation centers, and also expanded to other relevant governmental sectors beyond medical institutions [3].

The following text will focus on the key processes of OD and elaborate on the required multidisciplinary expertise and the involvement of multidisciplinary professional teams.

2.2.1 Identification and referral of potential donors

The clinical procedure of OD begins with the identification of potential donors. The potential donor identification rate determines the total scale of organs for transplantation [8]. Identification of potential donor and referral by the health care team to the OPO should occur in a timely manner. A timely referral is built upon a working mechanism of OD within donor hospitals with OPO [9]. In the United States (US), in addition to the fact that Centers for Medicare and Medicaid Services (CMS) require each imminent death should be referred by hospitals to the OPO for assessment, OPO will sign a contract with every single donor hospital in its donation service area to consolidate such partnership [10]. In the Netherlands, the roles of emergency physicians, neurosurgeons, and neurologists were clearly defined for the identification of potential organ donors [11]. In China, the health authority has included the potential donor reporting rate as one of the key performance indicators in the accreditation of third-grade hospitals [12].

In addition, research results have illustrated the importance of the ICU team's attitudes and recognition toward OD, as well as the active participation in OD to improve OD rate and organ procurement efficiency [13, 14]. Spanish recommendation even advocates that intensive care to facilitate OD (ICOD) is a legitimate practice that should be considered as part of the health care service portfolio of any country that has a regulated OD and OT system [15].

2.2.2 Death determination

All OD cases must strictly adhere to the internationally recognized ethical principle of "Dead Donor Rule". Either neurological or circulatory standards are adopted in death determination, such clinical practice has to be performed in accordance with local clinical protocols and legal and ethical requirements.

Although there exists global variability in brain death (BD) diagnosis, donation after brain death (DBD) still represents the main organ source of transplantation, accounting for 77.2% of global deceased donation in 2019 [5]. In this chapter, we focus on the BD determination.

Various protocols and guidelines for BD diagnosis have made clear requirements on the clinical criteria, operational specifications, and personnel for determining BD [16]. As for "who can certify", the World Brain Death Project report [17] provides a minimum recommendation. The physician performing the BD determination must be certified to practice medicine and trained in BD diagnosis. The determination team needs to include a neurologist, a neurosurgeon, an anesthesiologist, and an intensivist at least.

Although personnel in charge of OD and OT cannot take part in the process of death determination, whether the BD diagnosis can be carried out in a timely manner may have impacts on the subsequent step of the OD procedure and result in the donor loss. Thus, it can be seen that the support of neurological expertise and the involvement of a team specialized in performing BD determination are indispensable in this critical aspect of death determination.

2.2.3 Evaluation and maintenance of potential donors and organs

Potential donor evaluation is one of the key parts of OD workflow, which includes clinical assessment of the donor and organ viability, as well as the risk assessment of the donation process.

Clinical assessment involves risk assessment of donor-driven infectious disease to recipients and assessment of organ viability [18]. For detection of malignancies, it is necessary to know whether the donor has a history of malignancy diagnosis, chemotherapy, and surgery [19]. As for screening of infectious diseases, viral infections such as hepatitis, herpes, human polyomavirus, and acute neoplastic virus; bacterial infections such as acute infections, bacterial sepsis, meningitis, pulmonary infections, urinary tract infections, and multidrug resistant bacteria; and other pathogenic infections such as fungal infections, parasitic protozoan, and nematode infections, and prions need to be included [20]. In the case of evaluating elderly or marginal donors, cooperation between OPO medical specialists and transplant surgeons with extensive experience is needed. The entire medical evaluation also requires the professional support from the fields of laboratory medicine, infection, oncology, medical imageology, and pathology.

The other part of the evaluation process includes a general review of personal, social, and medical information of the potential donor as well as information regarding his/her family status and next of kin. The transplant coordinators need to screen and analyze risk points at hand and seek professional help from ethical and legal experts, social workers, and religious figures, if necessary.

Donor management is the longest-lasting step of the entire process and one of the key factors affecting the quality of organs and the transplant outcome [21]. ICU specialists have the professional advantage of carrying out donor maintenance thanks to their background and clinical experience [22]. Studies indicate that the engagement of ICU medical staff in donor management with an aggressive approach can improve the organ utilization rate and organ quality [23].

2.2.4 Communication with the family of the potential donor

As one of the core steps in OD procedure, family communication is considered a serious and professional matter. The family's distrust of the communicator and the content of the conversation is one of the major reasons for the refusal to donate. The family trust is built upon continuous communication and empathy demonstrated by the communicators. Effective communication with the donor's family requires knowledge reserves of medicine, ethics, law, psychology, social humanities, narrative medicine, communication, etc., close cooperation between coordinators and the health care team, as well as timely coordination among sectors such as traffic police, the forensic team, airlines company, civil affairs, and funeral institutions [24].

In addition to providing families with professional advices in a respectful, honest, cooperative, and empathetic manner during the process, psychological knowledge is needed to grasp the fluctuating psychological state of the family. Communication about death diagnosis and medical condition requires professional medical knowledge and then needs to be transferred to the family in an easy-to-understand way with communication skills. At the same time, traditional cultural and religious views also influence their willingness to donate to some extent. Positive arguments of traditional culture and religion on OD need to be invoked to guide the family to make appropriate decisions based on respecting their religious and cultural beliefs [24].

2.2.5 Organ allocation

Although organ allocation policies vary among countries in detail, all of them are based on the principle of fairness, equity, and transparency. The WHO guiding principles require that the allocation of organs, cells, and tissues should be guided by clinical criteria and ethical norms, not financial considerations [7]. The WMA Statement on Organ and Tissue Donation (The WMA Statement) regulates those policies governing the management of waiting lists should ensure efficiency and fairness [25]. Therefore, to balance the gains and losses posed by different dimensions, the research and development of organ allocation policies should be conducted by a panel of experts in multiple fields such as transplantation medicine, biomedicine, health economics, public health, statistics, ethics, law, etc.

To ensure the implementation of organ allocation is inconsistent with the targeted manner and adheres to the predefined allocation rules, the calculation of the matching list and the allocation processes afterward shall be carried out via an informative system [6]. Unlike any other data registries, the informative system for organ allocation has specific application characteristics such as faithful implementation of allocation policies, and real-time assistance in clinical decision-making. The design, development, and maintenance of the allocation system require a panel of medical experts as well as technical support of professionals in mathematics, information science, and computer science.

2.2.6 Organ procurement and preservation

A sound and reliable process of organ procurement, preservation, and transportation can improve the utilization of donated organs, and ensure the safety of the recipients [26]. According to the EU Guidelines on Quality and Safety of Transplanted Organs (6th edition) (The EU Guidelines) [27], a joint-effort approach among OPO, the donor hospitals, and the surgical team is required. In addition, the importance of establishing a specialized organ surgical team is emphasized in the EU Guidelines, which, if possible, shall consist of surgeons specializing in abdominal and cardiopulmonary organ retrieval, physician for anesthesia, and technicians responsible for organ perfusion preservation [27].

2.2.7 Education and publicity

Studies suggest that donation rates can be effectively increased through various types of campaigns for different targeted groups [28]. The WMA statement indicates that public awareness of OD should be raised through multifaceted and multilevel media awareness and public campaigns [25]. Through long-term and effective social publicity, it is expected to gradually create a favorable cultural and social atmosphere for OD.

Multilevel and multichannel popularization and publicity require strict standards and the guidance of communication knowledge, which itself is a multidisciplinary integration of narrative medicine, sociology, psychology, journalism, and communication. The promotion of OD requires the participation of ambassadors of OPOs, medical practitioners, media workers, educators, volunteers, and university (medical) students, etc.

2.3 Improvement of operational efficiency and service quality requires the support of multidisciplinary and multi-team professionals

The "conversion rate" is considered a key indicator to measure the professionalism and performance of the involved teams in the OD process. The "conversion rate" refers to the number of actual donors over the total number of potential donors, which is in contrast to the proportion of donor loss. The "critical pathway for deceased organ donation" systematically describes 13 common causes of donor loss (**Table 1**) [9]. In addition to objective factors (e.g., patients with contraindications

Systematical reasons	Fail to identify/refer potential donors
	Fail to confirm death determination
	Fail to declare circulatory system death within the appropriate time
	Logistical problems
	No suitable recipients
Donor or donor organs reasons	Medical examination does not meet the requirements (with contraindication to organ donation)
	Hemodynamic instability/unexpected cardiac arrest
	Anatomical, histological, and/or functional abnormalities of organs
	Organ damage during repair
	Inadequate organ perfusion or thrombosis
Reasons for permission/informed consent (communication issues)	The deceased explicitly declined to become a donor during lifetime
	Donor's family refusal to organ donation
	The forensic coroner or other judicial officer does not agree to organ donation

Table 1.
Reasons why potential donors do not become actual donors (donor loss causes).

to OD), some of these causes are related to the level of awareness and expertise of practitioners engaged in different steps along the process. These causes of donor loss can be improved by providing professional training to practitioners. But it is further illustrated here that potential donors cannot be converted into actual donors or the organ quality and the rights of recipients cannot be protected without the support of relevant expertise and the involvement of professional teams.

3. OD discipline built upon multidisciplinary integration

The construction of discipline includes building of theoretical system, carriers, talent training and career path, academic environment, and scientific research innovation.

3.1 Building of theoretical system

The multidisciplinary integration of OD discipline is reflected at two levels, which is firstly reflected in the integration of knowledge in the area within the medical domain (transplantation medicine, critical care medicine, neurology, infection, oncology, and pathology). The second level of multidisciplinary integration is the integration of knowledge in the area of law, ethics, public health, humanities, health economics, management, psychology and communication, etc. [3]. The multidisciplinary knowledge base supporting multi-team collaborative practice meets the fundamental needs of the construction of OD discipline.

3.2 Building of carriers

Although management models used in different countries vary, administrative organizations at all levels for OD and OT, donor hospitals, OPOs are practice bases of OD discipline.

The essence of multidisciplinary-supporting in OD practice indicates that effort should not only be paid for the construction of any single carrier for OD program with high operating efficiency but also for the long-term work collaboration mechanism between carriers. In the OD context, a collaboration mechanism means an efficient network of collaborations, at the institutional level, between community, OPO, medical institutions, hospice institutes, relevant government sectors, charities, and academic organizations, as well as at the individual level, volunteers, social workers, ICU teams, coordinators, medical experts, transplantation teams, legal medical experts, undertakers, scientific researchers, and other professionals.

3.3 Path of talent training and professional development

The building of the OD discipline requires the active engagement of multidisciplinary professionals and needs to train a host of application-oriented composite professionals and make them the main force for driving the development of the field.

A transplant coordinator is a profession derived from the development of the OD program and is key to promoting multi-team coordination and cooperation in the process of OD [29]. As the work of OD coordinators involves many aspects, efforts shall be made to strengthen their multidisciplinary theoretical reserve and develop their comprehensive abilities. Meanwhile, coordinators in different countries vary in their professional background, employer, requirements on qualification review, performance management system, etc. Actions should be taken to effectively utilize local occupational planning and policies on talent training, arrange and establish an appropriate professional development path and a system of occupational promotion for OD coordinators, and establish corresponding knowledge, ability, and technology training system in accordance with different features and work needs in different stages of career development. These actions are the fundamental guarantee for the continuous growth of the OD talent team and the basic guarantee for steady development of local OD [29].

3.4 Academic environment and scientific research innovation

In terms of creating a favorable academic environment, specialized international and national/regional associations related to OD have been created, and their members are experts and scholars in emergency and critical care medicine, neurology, OPO, transplantation medicine, oncology, ethics, law, medical humanities, hospital management, communication, sociology, health economics, public health management statistics, etc.

These associations regularly launch academic research and activities participated by multiple parties, produce high-quality scientific publications, guidelines, and expert consensuses related to organ and tissue donation, organize and take part in multidisciplinary forums and offline academic seminars, so as to create a favorable academic environment for building the OD multi-discipline system and continuously promote the professional development of OD.

The common research goals in OD-related scientific research tasks include how to maximize the outcomes linked to the mission of the OD program. These key indicators include the donor per million population (PMP), the donor conversion rate, authorization rate, the organ utilization rate, the degree of efficiency of the management mode and the collaborative network, and satisfaction of donor's family or relevant practitioners. The involvement of multi-discipline teams in these researches enhances the ability to find comprehensive solutions to the questions concerned. With regard to technical innovation, recent years have seen the development of technologies such as regional perfusion, ex vivo perfusion, mechanical preservation, and tissue regeneration to provide better conditions for organ viability and quality. Advances in biochemistry and tissue engineering have provided technical support to improve the quality and utilization of donor organs. Besides, with the development of aeronautical engineering technology, the concept of organ transportation by unmanned aircraft systems has been put into practice [3], indicating the enormous potential and value brought by the "medical + engineering + information" integration in the process of building of the OD discipline.

4. China's efforts

Over the past decade, China has made breakthroughs in OD and OT. Since the launch of the national program for deceased OD in 2010 and continuously driven by the patients' demands for transplantation, China has formed a national ethical OD and OT system in line with WHO guidelines and international standards [3]. China has become the second largest country in the world in terms of an annual number of OD and OT [5]. As of August 2022, the number of deceased organ donors has exceeded 40,000, and over 120,000 organs have been donated for saving life [30].

However, similar to other countries, China is still faced with the huge gap between supply and demand for OT. Meanwhile, China's PMP, 3.6 in 2020, is globally at the middle level [5], indicating room for improvement. The lack of a complete scientific theoretical system to guide professional and career development in OD is one of the reasons for the current results, rather than Asian or traditional cultures. In addition, the current number of transplant coordinators in China is insufficient, with around 2,000 certified coordinators [3] serving a population of 1.4 billion. Actions should be taken to implement countermeasures of talent attraction and talent encouragement for the field. To study and solve bottleneck problems facing the country, the work team consisting of multidisciplinary experts has made a proposal and reached a consensus on promoting OD discipline building through multidisciplinary integration and support.

4.1 Policy support

In recent years, China has advocated the development strategy of interdisciplinary collaboration and introduced a raft of policies, making multidisciplinary penetration and integration of interdisciplinary professionals a general trend [31]. Moreover, Chinese laws and regulations related to OD and OT advocate that administrative departments, red cross societies, and medical institutions at all levels and medical professionals shall support and take an active part in the work of OD. The introduction of these policies provides multidisciplinary integration and development of OD with institutional support [32, 33].

4.2 Tasks and actions

4.2.1 Building of OPOs

The degree of specialization of the operating carrier and its talent team is the basis for maintaining the efficient operation of the OD system. In 2013, advocated by the national health commission, China started building of OPOs nationwide [34], which, together with donor hospitals, become the carriers and initial base for the practice of the OD discipline. Subsequently, more than 130 OPOs have been developed either in a hospital-based or an independent institutional structure [35]. The standards for building, operation, and management of OPO and the indicators matrix of quality control for organ procurement have been also released by the national health commission [34].

4.2.2 Building of talent team

For the talent development of OD, the multidisciplinary knowledge and skill enhancement of professionals have been emphasized in its training model and contents in recent years. China has been exploring educational models for different target groups in practice, and the talent training includes the following aspects:

At the national level, comprehensive training courses and qualification tests are provided by China OD administration center for transplant coordinators, forming a national training and qualification system.

At the regional level, professional training is conducted by academic associations and OPOs for medical and nursing staff of critical care units, as well as public charity publicity and education activities for communities, schools, nursing homes, etc.

In terms of linking with the educational system, China has made explorations and practices in integrating education related to OD in the higher education system. The China-Europe Knowledge Transfer and Leadership in Organ Donation (KeTLOD) has established OD higher education (postgraduate) programs in seven Chinese universities to provide a master's course on organ donation [36]. In addition, a number of universities and colleges have introduced undergraduate elective courses on OD and OT [37]. In regions such as Zhejiang province, "popular science articles regarding OD " has been included in secondary school textbooks to popularize relevant concepts [38].

4.2.3 Academic environment

At the academic level, China has established professional associations for OD, which consist of medical experts from departments related to OD and OT, as well as scholars from medical ethics, law, social humanities, health economics, psychology, mass communication, biological tissue engineering, and anatomy. An expert consensus on development of a multidisciplinary supporting system for OD has been reached. Under the supervision of these associations, the scientific papers, consensus, guidelines, and books focused on the theme of multidisciplinary integration have been published, and academic activities with the participation of experts from multiple fields have been organized on a regular basis.

4.3 Social engagement

In terms of public education and publicity of OD, from the public-welfare publicity activities initiated by the administrative department, news media, and various public-service organizations to individual's spontaneous publicity activities, the concept of OD has been popularized. April has been granted as the memorial month for organ donors in the country. As of August 2022, the number of voluntary organ donor registrants in China has exceeded 4.9 million [30].

5. Conclusion

The construction of the OD discipline system is in line with the fundamental requirement of promoting sustainable development of OD and OT. Promoting the OD discipline development is of positive significance for enhancing the professional identity of OD practitioners and the credibility of the OD undertaking.

According to its attribute of public welfare and work characteristics of the OD undertaking, its disciplinary building needs interdisciplinary support. Through years of efforts, China has been improving relevant laws and regulations, besides, it strives to boost interdisciplinary collaboration of OD through diversified popularization and publicity, comprehensive training for professional teams, and creation of a collaborative network with more extensive multidisciplinary support and engagement.

In summary, whether to cope with the bottleneck problems in the development of OD, or to improve the efficiency of work system and the quality of medical services by taking key measures to meet the demands in the whole process, it shows the necessity and feasibility of promoting the building of OD-related disciplines through multidisciplinary collaboration. Therefore, under the strategy of multidisciplinary development, we need to center around safeguarding the rights of donors and their family members and protecting recipients' rights to health, focus on the quality of the work of OD and OT, effectively integrate resources, give full play to professional forces in different fields, build an OD discipline system that meets the professional medical requirements, and fully shows the features of social humanity, thereby promoting the standardized, systematic, and professional development of OD. It is a common topic requiring policymakers, experts, and practitioners in the field to think deeply and make research, explorations, and practices persistently. We believe, by adhering to the coordinated multidisciplinary development strategy, the visible progress of the organ donation discipline in the future would be the result of the joint-effort gained from interdisciplinary collaboration and innovations.

Acknowledgements

We would like to express our special thanks to the National Health Commission of China and the Red Cross Society of China for their administrative support in establishing the national program of deceased organ donation & transplantation and the development of a data collection system. We would like to extend our sincere gratitude to the pioneers in the field including Prof Jiefu HUANG, Prof Bingyi SHI, Prof Shusen ZHENG, Prof Yongfeng LIU, Mr. Fengzhong HOU, etc. for their professional leadership in the reform of the Chinese organ transplantation in the last 10 years. Appreciation is also given to the Shanxi Provincial Organ Procurement and Allocation Center for logistics support of the study.

Funding

There has been no dedicated funding for this study.

Conflict of interest

The authors declare no conflict of interest.

Author details

Wenshi Jiang[1*], Xiaotong Wu[1], Liansheng Ma[2], Jing Shu[3], Juan Yan[4], Liming Yang[5], Yajie Ma[1] and Xiangxiang He[1]

1 Shanxi Provincial Organ Procurement and Allocation Center, Taiyuan, China

2 First Hospital of Shanxi Medical University, Taiyuan, China

3 Zhejiang Xin'an International Hospital, Hangzhou, China

4 Shanxi Medical University, School of Humanities and Social Sciences, Taiyuan, China

5 The Sixth Hospital of Shanxi Medical University, Taiyuan, China

*Address all correspondence to: wenshi.jiang@hotmail.com

References

[1] Wang Z, Peng D, Ma X. From interdisciplinarity to interdisciplinarity: The case of the United States and its insights. Science Bulletin. 2021;**66**(9):9

[2] Xue Z, Zhang Z. A review of interdisciplinary research systems. Library and Information Work. 2020;**64**(14):14

[3] Professional Committee of Human Organ and Tissue Donation, China Association for the Promotion of Human Health Science and Technology. Organ donation: A new multidisciplinary discipline in China in the new era. Organ Transplantation. 2020;**11**(5):614-621. DOI: 10.3969/j.issn.1674-7445.2020.05.015

[4] Rudge C, Matesanz R, Delmonico FL, et al. International practices of organ donation. British Journal of Anaesthesia. 2012;**1**(1):20

[5] GODT. Global observatory on donation and transplantation. 2022. Available from: http://www.transplant-observatory.org/. [Accessed: July 14, 2022]

[6] Huirui L. Why does the system fail? -- Research on the justice of organ donation distribution under multiple logics. Sociological Research. 2020;**1**:26

[7] Noel L. WHO guiding principles on human cell, tissue and organ transplantation. Transplantation. 2010;**90**(3):229-233

[8] Dong J, Xuyang L, Wang H, et al. Interpretation of guide to the quality and safety of organs for transplantation: Identification and referral of potential donors. Organ Transplantation. 2020;**11**(3):395-399. DOI: 10.3969/j.issn.1674-7445.2020.03.013

[9] The critical pathway for deceased donation: Reportable uniformity in the approach to deceased donation. Transplant Multinational. 2015;**4**:24

[10] Ehrle R. Timely referral of potential organ donors. Critical Care Nurse. 2006;**26**(2):88-93

[11] Witjes M, Kotsopoulos A, Otterspoor L, et al. The implementation of a multidisciplinary approach for potential organ donors in the emergency department. Transplantation. 2019;**103**:2060

[12] National Health Commission of the People's Republic of China. Evaluation criteria for tertiary hospitals (2020 version). (EB/QL). 2020

[13] Roels L, Spaight C, Smits J, et al. Critical care staffs' attitudes, confidence levels and educational needs correlate with countries' donation rates: Data from the Donor Action Database. Transplantation International. 2010;**23**(8):842-850

[14] Fang Q, Wu XL, Wang F. Organ donation and critical care medicine. Chinese Medical Journal. 2019;**99**(35):4

[15] Martín-Delgado MC, Martínez-Soba F, Masnou N, et al. Summary of Spanish recommendations on intensive care to facilitate organ donation. Chinese Medical Journal. 2019;**19**:1782-1791

[16] Shemie SD, Hornby L, Baker A, et al. International guideline development for the determination of death. Intensive Care Medicine. 2014;**6**:40

[17] Greer DM, Shemie SD, Lewis A, et al. Determination of brain death/death

by neurologic criteria: The world brain death project[J]. Jama. 2020;**324**(11): 1078-1097

[18] Xie L, Qiuxiang X, Xianpeng Z, et al. Interpretation of Guide to the Quality and Safety of Organs for Transplantation: Evaluation and selection criteria for donors and organs. Organ Transplantation. 2020;**11**(4):487-491. DOI: 10.3969/j.issn.1674-7445.2020.04.011

[19] Lin J, Shixin L, Yang Y. Interpretation of guide to the quality and safety of organs for transplantation: Risk of malignant tumor transmission. Organ Transplantation. 2020;**11**(3): 400-404. DOI: 10.3969/j.issn.1674-7445.2020.03.014

[20] Bogen Y, Lei Z. Interpretation of guild to the quality and safety of organs for transplantation: Risk of infectious disease transmission. Organ Transplantation. 2020;**11**(2): 282-287. DOI: 10.3969/j.issn.1674-7445.2020.02.016

[21] Sun X, Dong J, Qin K, et al. Optimizing donor clinical management strategies and promoting scientific research on donor management. Organ Transplantation. 2019;**10**(6):731-734. DOI: 10.3969/j.issn.1674-7445.2019.06.018

[22] Pan A, Wang P, Xie C, et al. A key strategy for ICU-assisted organ donation as a relay for life. Organ Transplantation. 2020;**11**(2):288-292. DOI: 10.3969/j.issn.1674-7445.2020.02.017

[23] Zhu Y, Cai C, Guan X. Donor management of organ donation in ICU. Chinese Electronic Journal of Intensive Care Medicine. 2017;**3**(2):6

[24] Preparation Group of Expert Consensus on Communication with Families of Organ and Tissue Donors. Expert consensus on communication with families of organ and tissue donors. Organ Transplantation. 2021;**12**(6):651-661. DOI: 10.3969/j.issn.1674-7445.2021.06.003

[25] World Medical Association. WMA Statement on Organ and Tissue Donation [EB/OL]. 2020. Available from: https://www.wma.net/policies-post/wma-statement-on-organ-and-tissue-donation/

[26] Huibo S, Wang X, Xu J, et al. Interpretation of guide to the quality and safety of organs for transplantation: Organ procurement, preservation and transportation. Organ Transplantation. 2020;**11**(2):276-281. DOI: 10.3969/j.issn.1674-7445.2020.02.015

[27] European Committee (Partial Agreement) on Organ Transplantation (CD-P-TO) EDQM. Guidelines on the Quality and Safety of Transplant Organs. 6th ed. Beijing: Science Publishers; 2019;**6**(2)

[28] Madden S, Lucey MR, Neuberger J. Does publicity affect organ donation? Transplant International. 2020;**33**:1146-1148

[29] Yang S, Xiaoqin T, Gao X, et al. Consideration on the professional construction of organ donation coordinator team. China Journal of Transplantation. 2012;**6**(2)

[30] China Organ Donation Administrative Center. Available from: https://www.codac.org.cn. [Accessed: August 2, 2022]

[31] Academic Degrees Committee of China State Council. Notice on the Issuance of the Measures for the Establishment and Management of Interdisciplinary Subjects (for Trial

Implementation) [A/OL]. 2022. Available from: http://www.gov.cn/xinwen/2021-12/06/content_5656041.htm

[32] Law of the People's Republic of China on the Red Cross Society (revised 2017) [EB/OL]. 2022. Available from: http://www.npc.gov.cn/npc/c12435/201702/5cbcc78a701b4a8dbf3bd0a6701659e2.shtml

[33] General Committee of the Red Cross Society of China, National Health and Wellness Commission. Notice on the issuance of the Measures for the Administration of Human Organ Donation Coordinators [A/OL]. 2022. Available from: https://www.redcross.org.cn/html/2021-05/78447.html

[34] Huang W, Ye QF, Fan XL, et al. Development and history of organ procurement organization in China. Medical Journal. 2021;**42**(2):173-178

[35] Jiang W et al. The first independent provincial OPO in China: The Shanxi Experience. Transplantation. 2022;**106**(6):1093-1095

[36] China-Europe Organ Donation Leadership Training and Expertise Transfer Program, Jiang WS, Ballester C. Exploration and practice of a higher education model for organ donation. Chinese Journal of Transplantation. 2019;**13**(3):201-205

[37] Ling S-B, Chen J-L, Wei Q, et al. The impact of general education on organ donation and organ transplantation on improving humanistic literacy of college students. China Higher Medical Education. 2021;**5**:2

[38] China Human Organ Donation Management Center. Human organ donation knowledge into high school textbooks in Zhejiang Province. 2022. Available from: https://www.codac.org.cn/contentdon/work_dynamics/20220104/1030335092.html. [Accessed: January 04, 2022]

Section 2

Ethical and Religious Issues in Organ Donation

Chapter 3

Altruistic Kidney Donation: Overview and Ethical Considerations

Kudirat Busari and Abigail Garba

Abstract

End-stage kidney disease is a global pandemic which exerts significant morbidity, mortality as well as economic burden on affected patients. Kidney transplantation, either from cadaveric or living donors, offers the best therapeutic choice to improve survival and quality of life. However, due to the increasing prevalence of end-stage kidney disease, there is a great mismatch between the demand and supply of donor organs. Efforts to mitigate this dire shortage include altruistic organ donations. Altruistic donation refers to organ donation by an individual who is neither genetically nor emotionally related to the potential recipient. This concept at its inception received a lot of resistance from the transplant community and continues to raise ethical concerns. This chapter reviews altruistic organ donation, ethical considerations and its potential benefits.

Keywords: altruistic donation, end-stage kidney disease, ethical considerations, kidney transplantation, living kidney donations, non-directed donors

1. Introduction

End-stage kidney disease (ESKD) is associated with life-threatening complications which have significant adverse impact on both the affected individual and the health-care system [1]. Kidney transplantation remains the favored therapeutic option for improving survival and quality of life, and reducing morbidity in patients with ESKD [1]. Transplantation can be either from deceased donors or living donors [1].

Living kidney donor transplantation, which can either be directed (related) or non-directed (unrelated), has been demonstrated to have superior recipient and graft outcomes compared to cadaveric donation [2]. In addition, living kidney donors form an important link filling the gap of significant donor organ shortage that leads to prolonged waitlist times. In 2014, according to data from the Organ Procurement Transplantation Network (OPTN), over 4000 individuals on the waitlist died while waiting for a kidney transplantation while an additional 3668 became unfit for the rigors of transplantation. Similarly, the United States Renal Data System estimates that the average waitlist time is 3.6 years [3–5].

Altruistic donation, a form of living kidney donation, has been referred to by many terms in literature including: non-directed donation (American terminology), unspecified donation (European), Good Samaritan donation and anonymous donation [6, 7]. It is a fairly recent development which is rapidly gaining popularity in these times [6–8]. According to the Cambridge English Dictionary, altruism can be defined as the "willingness to do things that bring advantages to others, even if it results in disadvantage for yourself" [9]. In transplant medicine, altruistic donors are donors who are neither genetically nor emotionally related to the potential transplant recipients i.e. donation to a virtual stranger [7, 10, 11]. This definition, which implies no obvious benefits to the donor, is perhaps one of the reasons why much skepticism abounds about this form of organ donation [6, 7]. The road to altruistic organ donation has been paved with many stumbling stones borne from scandals and individual reluctance of transplant surgeons and community non-acceptance [6–8].

2. History of living kidney donation and altruistic donation

Living kidney donation has been in existence for almost seven decades, since an identical twin donated to his brother in 1954 at the Peter Brent Brigham hospital in Boston; it has progressively increased in practice following immense strides in surgical techniques and immunosuppressive therapy [12]. It now accounts for up to one-third of transplants in both the United Kingdom (UK) and United States (US) and the entirety of transplants in many African and Middle-Eastern countries [6, 7].

The first report of altruistic kidney donation occurred in the US in the seventies when Sadler *et al.*, reported a series of 30 living unrelated kidney transplant recipients [13]. However, interest in this practice waned due to the relatively low success rates of transplantation from genetically unrelated donors at this time [13]. This was coupled with a number scandals in the eighties involving commercial organ procurement and transplant tourism; this sparked ethical debates and led to the advent of the National Organ Transplant Act (NOTA) in 1984 which expressly prohibited the purchase of donor organs [8, 14–16]. However, at the turn of the millennium, there was a resurgence in altruistic donation when Matas *et al.* reported success with 22 kidney transplant recipients [17]. Since then, it has progressively gained popularity, with over 3900 altruistic donations taking place in the US from 2001 till date (representing >2% of all living kidney donations) and this number is expected to increase [5, 10, 18]. In fact, according to data from the Organ Procurement and Transplantation Network, an all-time high record of 476 anonymous kidney donors was reported in 2021 and another 194 by June 2022 (**Figure 1**) [18].

In the UK, the Human Organ Transplant Act of 1989 criminalized transplantation in genetically unrelated donor-recipient pairs unless they were formally approved by the Unrelated Live Transplantation Regulatory Authority and altruistic donation was discouraged [11]. However, the Human Tissue Act and Human Tissue Authority, which came into legislation in 2004 and 2006 respectively, enabled altruistic kidney donation to commence; similar to the US experience, its incidence has increased, with majority of transplant centres partaking, and now accounting for 80 to 110 transplants per year [6, 11, 14]. Altruistic kidney donation now takes place in several countries including US, UK, Netherlands, Canada, Australia, Sweden and Spain, with the majority occurring in the former three regions [7]. **Figure 2** is a bar chart depicting the increasing incidence of altruistic kidney donation in the UK [6].

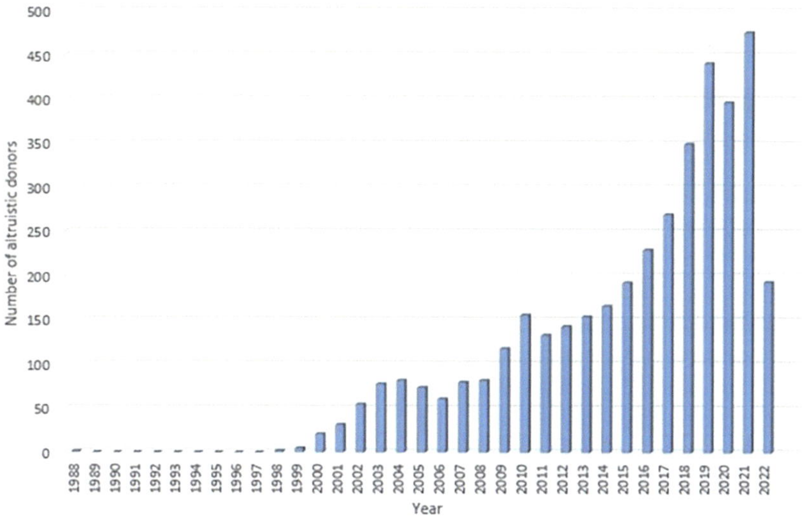

Figure 1.
Bar chart depicting the number of living non-biological unrelated anonymous donations per year in the US. Bar chart based on data culled from: Donor: Living donor relation to recipient by donation year. Organ procurement and transplantation network [internet]. Available from: http://www.optn.transplant.hrsa.gov. [accessed: 2022-2107-31].

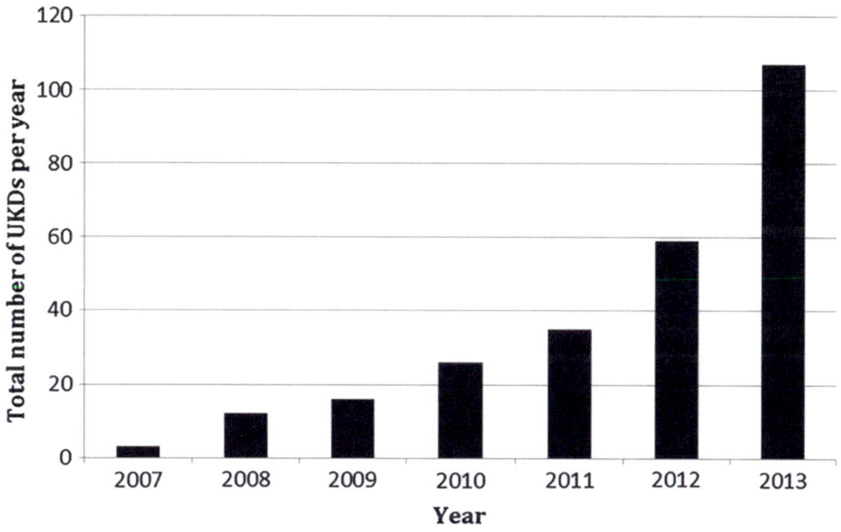

Figure 2.
Bar chart depicting the number of unspecified kidney donations (UKD) occurring per year in the UK. Source: [6].

3. Altruistic kidney donation

The premise of altruistic kidney donation has raised a lot of questions such as "What is the driving force behind altruistic organ donation?" and "What does the altruistic organ donor gain from such an endeavour?" [19]. However, since it is a viable source of kidney allograft, the transplant physician should be conversant with the factors that limit its acceptance and the guidelines and ethical considerations pertaining to its practice. These issues will be addressed in the following sub-sections:

3.1 Characteristics of the altruistic donor

In literature, the description of the altruistic donor is non-specific; however, in the study by Kumar *et al.*, it was reported that altruistic donors were more likely to be females and Caucasian in origin [20]. In other studies, they were also predominantly Caucasian, older (averagely 10 years older than directed donors), retirees with religious inclinations and often had previous surgical procedures [6, 21]. They also tended not to have active dependents and were more involved in other altruistic endeavors such as volunteerism, blood donation, monetary charity, etc [6, 20, 21].

3.2 Motives of the altruistic donor

This has been the source of many debates in the transplant community. Without apparent direct benefits and with added potential surgical risks, what drives the altruistic donor? [19, 22]. It is therefore understandable that many transplant physicians regard this altruism with skepticism and shun the practice. Studies have shown that the primary motivation for altruistic donation arises from a pressing desire to be of help, a strong sense of empathy and the inclination that the benefits to the recipient outweigh the personal risks incurred. Many of these donors have a heightened sense of moral obligation, but secondary gains such as time off work, media attention or popularity may be additional inciting factors [6, 7, 22, 23]. Since most of these individuals are often already involved in other altruistic endeavors, it is not far-fetched if extended to living organ donation.

3.3 Guidelines for altruistic kidney donation

There are no standardized, globally-accepted guidelines or policies underlying the process of altruistic kidney donation [8, 10, 16, 24]. Regardless of individual transplant centre practices, any proposed guideline on altruistic donation should include the following core tenets:

- Mitigation of risks to the altruistic donor: This requires a rigorous and unbiased pre-donation evaluation process [8, 24].

- Avoidance of financial compensation: Financial compensation can be construed as undue inducement or coercion and still remains illegal in many countries [14, 15, 24].

- Maintenance of anonymity of the recipient-donor pair: Though difficult to attain, this protects the recipient from potential exploitation and an unrealistic sense of obligation, while protecting the donor from breach of privacy, anxiety about transplant outcomes, donation pressure and undue attention from the recipient, preserving the altruism of the act [23, 25]. To preserve anonymity, the University of Minnesota proposed registering the donors under aliases and admitting recipients and donors in different hospital wings; however, these measures are not infallible [3, 6, 24, 25]. Most countries insist on total anonymity for altruistic donation and this remains lifelong in Netherlands and Sweden;

however, the UK recently revoked this, allowing anonymity to be lifted 6 months after donation on request from both parties [3].

- Minimizing potential conflicts of interest in transplant programs: Conflicts of interest may arise when transplant programs involved in altruistic kidney donation are responsible for sourcing and allocating these organs to patients on their own waitlists. This may foster competitive pressure to improve performance at the expense of appropriate donor assessment [6, 14, 24].

3.3.1 Evaluation of the altruistic donor

Evaluation of the altruistic kidney donor often follows the same steps as the established process for living kidney donors with emphasis placed on additional psychological assessment by an independent certified psychiatrist/psychologist. Although the latter is no longer mandatory in the UK, it still remains standard practice [6, 8]. In the US, Crowley *et al.* [24] demonstrated in an analysis of 50 high-performance transplant centres and organ procurement organizations (OPO) that screening of the altruistic donor often follows five or six main steps:

1. A baseline screening interview: This often takes place over the phone between the intended altruistic donor and transplant physician. This provides preliminary medical history that can immediately rule out organ donation and ascertain the motives of the donor and his/her knowledge regarding the donation process [16, 24]. **Figure 3** below summarizes a proforma for this initial screening [16].

2. Provision of a comprehensive educational brochure to the altruistic donor.

3. In-person review: This is performed by the transplant physician and/or other team members and includes complete clinical history, physical examination, laboratory evaluation and obtaining informed consent.

4. Psychosocial evaluation: This is conducted by independent assessors including a behavioral scientist and/or a panel from the centre's transplant committee. This serves to protect the donor and ascertain his mental health. Some centres give a lag period after this assessment to allow the potential donor come to terms with his/her decision.

5. Donor nephrectomy and organ allocation: Allocation is done according to United Network for Organ Sharing and/or centre-specific clinical criteria in most centres while others use OPOs to facilitate organ distribution similar to cadaveric organs.

6. Post-donation review and monitoring: This follows the standard for living kidney donors but may not be ideal due to the peculiarities of this type of donor [7, 8, 10, 16, 20].

3.3.2 Models for altruistic kidney donation programs

Potential altruistic donors may influence how their organs are utilized. There are currently 2 models for altruistic donation programs [8, 11]:

TABLE 1. The initial screening interview

Medical/Personal History

- How old are you?
- Are you healthy and physically fit?
- Do you have a history of cancer, heart disease, diabetes, kidney disease, or high blood pressure?
- Do you take medications?
- Have you undergone any previous operations?
- Is there a history of kidney disease in your family?
- Do you receive disability benefits for any reason? (This does not rule out a donor a priori who should not be discouraged to proceed. They should be asked to elaborate.)
- Do you live alone? Are you married?
- Where do you live? (This will affect costs and convenience associated with donation.)

Knowledge About Nondirected Donation

- How did you learn or hear about organ donation?
- Do you understand that donating a kidney is not like donating blood?
- Are you aware that the risks of donating a kidney include the possibility of dying?
- Do you understand that there are risks to the recipient (i.e. that the kidney may be rejected)?
- Do you understand that you cannot be paid money for being a donor?
- Are you aware that several months may be necessary to determine your suitability as a donor by required clinical and psychological testing?
- Do you understand that you will not select your recipient and that he or she will be from the list of those who are already waiting?

Donor Related Questions

- Why do you wish to donate a kidney?
- Have you told a member of your family that you wish to be a kidney donor?
- Have you and your family considered the burdens associated with donation that could include out of pocket expenses for travel, doctor appointments, and time out of work?
- Is there a specific time frame to have your donor surgery performed?
- Would somebody be available to assist you at home during your recovery from surgery?

Figure 3.
Proforma depicting standard questions asked during the baseline interview between the altruistic donor and transplant Centre. Source: [16].

1. The donor organ may be included directly into the national transplant waitlist as previously done in most countries [8, 11].

2. Altruistic donations may be utilized in kidney sharing schemes, a more recent model that maximizes the number of transplantations. Kidney sharing schemes can be *paired donations* or *pooled altruistic donor chains* involving more than a pair of recipients. These schemes can occur simultaneously (so-called *domino donation chains*) or not (*non-simultaneous extended altruistic donor chains*) [8, 11]. Unfortunately, it may be time-consuming, involve a lot of logistics and increase the waitlist time for vulnerable recipients like the highly-sensitized one [8, 24]. **Figure 4** summarizes these models while **Figure 5** illustrates a kidney donation chain with the altruistic donor as the starting point [8, 11].

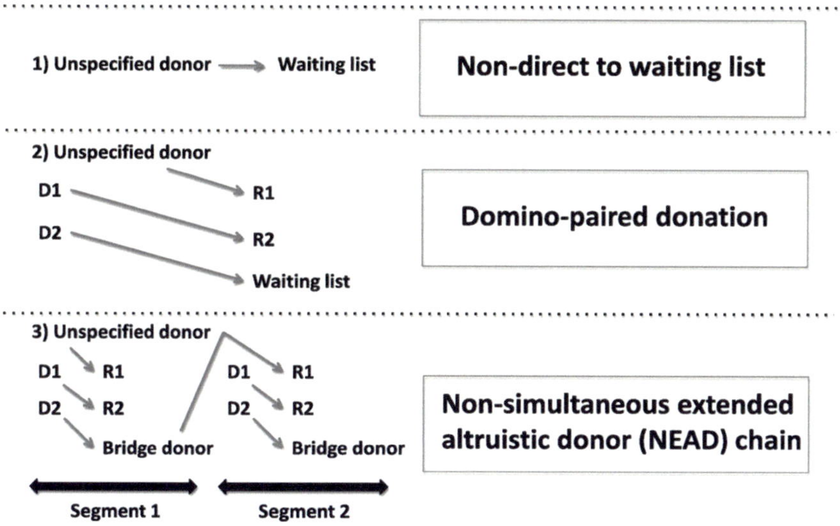

Figure 4.
Summary of altruistic donation models. D: Donor; R: Recipient. Source: [8].

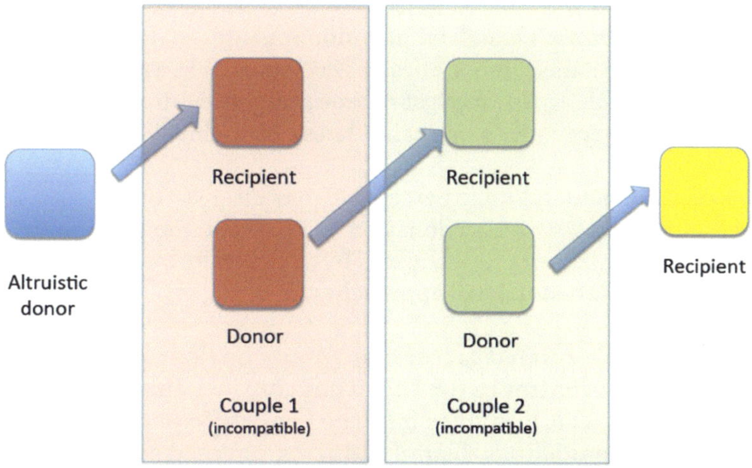

Figure 5.
Illustration of a pooled donation scheme with the altruistic donor at the fore-front. Source: [11].

3.4 Outcomes of altruistic kidney donation

There have been concerns about the outcomes, especially psychosocial, of altruistic donors [6–8, 10]. In a comparative study of the post-donation outcomes of altruistic donors versus directed donors over a 5-year period in the UK, Maple *et al.* reported no significant differences between the two cohorts across several psychosocial domains [6]. Furthermore, there were no differences in terms of post-operative outcomes such as duration of hospital stay, complication rates, incidence of hypertension and abnormal laboratory parameters [6]. However, the altruistic donors recovered faster post-operatively and returned earlier to their routine activities such as work (4–6 weeks *vs* 6–12 weeks, $p < 0.001$) and driving (<4 weeks *vs* 6–12 weeks, $p < 0.001$) [6]. This same study also assessed regret amongst the donors and found no significant differences in the degree of current or future regrets about organ donation [6]. Several small studies have reported outcomes comparable to Maple *et al.*'s findings [7, 21, 26].

Indirect benefits reported by altruistic donors include: improved self-esteem, augmented satisfaction with life, overall increased sense of wellbeing and a feeling that donation added extra meaning to their lives. Other secondary gains include work leave and media acclaim [6, 7].

On the other hand, adverse psychosocial outcomes of altruistic donation include difficulty obtaining health or life insurance, marital and familial conflicts, depression/anxiety disorders and loss of job or educational opportunities; these are not significantly different compared to directed donors and the general population [6, 7, 21, 26]. Similar to living donors, there may be an increased risk of post-donation hypertension (26.8%), surgical complications (1–10%) and peri-operative mortality (0.03%) [6, 7, 12].

3.5 Barriers to altruistic donation programs

Several barriers may prevent widespread use of altruistic donors:

- **Donor-related factors**: Though willing, donor health characteristics may limit their intent. For instance, donor obesity was reported in a study as a major cause (45%) of loss-to-follow-up amongst potential altruistic donors, and mental health concerns may render some candidates unsuitable [20].

- **Society-related factors**: Public perception may exaggerate the harm and safety concerns associated with organ donation and prevent interested individuals from stepping forward. This can be mitigated by appropriate awareness campaigns employing multiple educational approaches [3, 8, 10, 14].

- **Transplant centre-related factors**: In a study by Rodrigue *et al.* [8], up to 39% of transplant centres in the US do not consider altruistic donation as a viable option [8]. This hesitance is borne from different reasons including: lack of universal guidelines, fear of inducing physical and mental harm to the donors, concerns about the motives of altruistic donors, possibility of post-donation regrets, concerns that altruistic donation could lead to a decline in cadaveric donation, potential for litigation risks and potential requests for financial compensation leading to undue media attention [7, 24, 25, 27]. Some of these concerns are largely unsubstantiated and theoretical in nature [25, 27].

3.6 Ethical considerations for altruistic kidney donation

The concept of altruistic kidney donation has engendered many ethical issues which have slowed its acceptance and practice in the transplant community [27]. The concerns regarding some of the ethical principles are elucidated herein:

Beneficence: Since the primary obligation of the physician is to do no harm and protect patients, would altruistic donation not contradict the ethical principle of beneficence in relation to the donor even if it is at his own behest? Furthermore, as kidney transplantation is beneficial to patients with ESKD, would it be ethical to decline a potentially lifesaving procedure due to uncertainties about the motives of a potential altruistic donor? [8, 14, 16]. There are no simple answers to these questions but appropriate informed consent and pre-donation evaluation would ensure adequate protection of the donor. Additionally, laparoscopic donor nephrectomy minimizes the surgical risks borne by the donor.

Non-maleficence: The phrase "First do no harm" is one of the dictums that forms the bedrock of the modern practice of medicine. Is it then ethical for transplant physicians to actively solicit for altruistic donors? Although altruistic donation is potentially beneficial to a recipient, it may contravene the ethical principle of non-maleficence to the donor [8]. There have always been ethical concerns about exposing apparently-healthy individual to potential anesthetic and surgical risks. Some of these concerns have been partially allayed with advances in surgical techniques and post-operative care, improving donor safety.

Autonomy: Does rejecting altruistic donation contravene donor and recipient autonomy? Should the recipient reserve the right to reject or accept an organ from an altruistic donor? Is it paternalistic for transplant centres to arbitrarily refuse to evaluate such donors? [8, 14, 27]. While transplant physicians or nephrologists may be hesitant to accept kidneys from altruistic donors, they should only reject such organs on medical grounds after disclosure to the transplant recipients [8, 14]. Another ethical concern is pressure from the transplant centres on potential donors, especially in pooled donation schemes [8, 14]. This would be an indication to stop the process as it affects the ethical principle of donor autonomy [8, 14].

Justice: How do transplant programs maintain justice in the allocation of altruistic donor organs (i.e. distributive justice)? Who decides who benefits from altruistic donation, especially in the face of scarce donor organs? Some transplant centres prefer to channel such donations through a local OPO or national transplant waitlist to ensure justice, equitability and non-discrimination, as this reduces selection bias, allowing the recipient with the best compatibility to be transplanted [27].

Financial compensation: Should altruistic donors be offered financial compensation? Under the NOTA, it is acceptable to reimburse donors for minimal expenses incurred like medical bills, lost wages and transport fares [15, 27]. Excessive compensation is frowned upon, to avoid commercializing organ donation, prevent undue inducement of donors and protect the recipient from exploitation, blackmail and emotional distress [8, 14, 27, 28]. This is important because over 10% of global kidney transplantation occurs through organ trafficking and transplant tourism [27, 29]. In developing countries, patients pay out-of-pocket for renal replacement therapy and cadaveric donation is lacking, so commercialized transplantation is an open secret though illegal, and transplant tourism to procure donor organs is prevalent [14, 27,28]. This contrasts with the controversial Iranian model of compensated living unrelated kidney donation which has reduced waitlist times, with over half of ESKD patients having functional renal allografts [30, 31]. Some authors have proposed that incentivizing or regulating commercial organ donation may proffer a long-term solution to the scarcity of donor organs [32–34].

Other ethical considerations: Should donor-recipient pairs have contact in the peri-operative or post-donation period? While this may be beneficial, in some cases, it may foster unrealistic expectations of gratitude and indebtedness in the donor and may set him or her up for future disappointments [8, 27]. Unrelated living donation are considered less prone to subtle pressure and coercion as may occur in genetically or emotionally related donors [2, 16, 27, 28].

4. Conclusion

The practice of altruistic donation, although ethically controversial, has garnered success and popularity. The process is highly variable amongst individual transplant centres, leading to confusion, misconception and lack of motivation for interested individuals. Therefore, the process of donor evaluation, allocation and post-donation follow-up must be standardized globally. A rigorous evaluation protocol as well as mental health assessment and informed consent are imperative for successful implementation.

Advancing the practice of altruistic donation requires public awareness on the benefits of donation, donor risk minimization, advocacy and involvement of all relevant stakeholders. This procedure has the potential to increase transplantation rates and alleviate organ shortage and should hence be encouraged.

Acknowledgements

We acknowledge Professor Ahmed Halawa for his support.

Conflict of interest

The authors declare no conflict of interest.

Author details

Kudirat Busari[1,2]* and Abigail Garba[1]

1 Nisa Premier Hospital, Abuja, Nigeria

2 Institute of Medical Science, School of Medicine, University of Liverpool, United Kingdom

*Address all correspondence to: quarkim213@gmail.com

References

[1] Tonelli M, Wiebe N, Knoll G, et al. Systematic review: Kidney transplantation compared with dialysis in clinically relevant outcomes. American Journal of Transplantation. 2011;**11**(10):2093-2109

[2] Mendez R, Aswad S, Obispo E, et al. Extending organ availability with living-nonrelated renal transplants. In Transplantation Proceedings. 1992;**24**(5):2106-2107

[3] Mamode N, Lennerling A, Citterio F, et al. Anonymity and live-donor transplantation: An ELPAT view. Transplantation. 2013;**95**(4):536-541

[4] United States Renal Data System. Annual Data Report [Internet]. 2015. Available from: http://www.usrds.org [Accessed: May 12, 2022]

[5] U.S. Department of Health & Human Services Organ Procurement and Transplantation Network (OPTN) and Scientific Registry of Transplant Recipients (SRTR) Annual Report [Internet]. 2015. Available from: http://optn.transplant.hrsa.gov [Accessed: May 12, 2022]

[6] Maple H, Chilcot J, Burnapp L, et al. Motivations, outcomes, and characteristics of unspecified (non-directed altruistic) kidney donors in the United Kingdom. Transplantation. 2014;**98**(11):1182-1189

[7] Rodrigue JR, Schutzer ME, Paek M, Morrissey P. Altruistic kidney donation to a stranger: Psychosocial and functional outcomes at two US transplant centers. Transplantation. 2011;**91**(7):772-778

[8] Sharif A. Unspecified kidney donation - a review of principles, practice and potential. Transplantation. 2013;**95**(12):1425-1430

[9] Definition of Altruism. Cambridge Dictionary [Internet]. 2022. Available from: http://www.dictionary.cambridge.org/dictionary/english/altruism [Accessed: May 1, 2022]

[10] Kazley AS, Amarnath R, Palanisamy A, Taber D, Chavin K. Anonymous altruistic living kidney donation in the US: Reality and practice. International Journal of Transplantation Research Medicine. 2016;**2**:021

[11] Past and future of altruistic kidney donation [Internet]. 2022. Available from: http://www.giveakidney.org [Accessed: May 10, 2022]

[12] Bia MJ, Ramos EL, Danovitch GM, et al. Evaluation of living renal donors. The current practice of US transplant centers. Transplantation. 1995;**60**(4):322-327

[13] Sadler HH, Davison L, Carroll C, Kountz SL. The living, genetically unrelated, kidney donor. InSeminars in Psychiatry. 1971;**3**(1):86-101

[14] Ghods AJ. Ethical issues and living unrelated donor kidney transplantation. Iranian Journal of Kidney Diseases. 2009;**3**(4):183-191

[15] United States. National organ transplant act: Public law 98-507. US Statutes at Large. 1984;**98**:2339-2348

[16] Adams PL, Cohen DJ, Danovitch GM, et al. The non-directed live-kidney donor: Ethical considerations and practice guidelines: A National Conference Report. Transplantation. 2002;**74**(4):582-589

[17] Matas AJ, Garvey CA, Jacobs CL, Kahn JP. Non-directed donation of kidneys from living donors. NEJM. 2000;**343**(6):433-436

[18] Donor: Living donor relation to recipient by donation year. Organ Procurement and Transplantation Network Data Report [Internet]. Available from: http://www.optn.transplant.hrsa.gov [Accessed: July 31, 2022]

[19] Meran A. Organ donation: Altruism vs. incentive. AMA Journal of Ethics. 2002;**4**(8):235-237

[20] Kumar V, MacLennan P, Deierhoi R, et al. The altruistic living kidney donor phenotype-from inquiry to donation. Transplantation. 2018;**102**:S242

[21] Timmerman L, Zuidema WC, Erdman RA, Kranenburg LW, Timman R, et al. Psychologic functioning of unspecified anonymous living kidney donors before and after donation. Transplantation. 2013;**95**(11):1369-1374

[22] Balliet W, Kazley AS, Johnson E, et al. The non-directed living kidney donor: Why donate to strangers? Journal of Renal Care. 2019;**45**(2):102-110

[23] van den Bosch P. Non-directed altruistic kidney donation: A donor perspective. Journal of Renal Care. 2014;**40**(2):96-98

[24] Crowley-Matoka M, Switzer G. Non-directed living donation: A survey of current trends and practices. Transplantation. 2005;**79**(5):515-519

[25] Gewarges M, Poole J, De Luca E, et al. Canadian Society of Transplantation Members' views on anonymity in organ donation and transplantation. In Transplantation Proceedings. 2015;**47**(10):2799-2804

[26] Massey EK, Kranenburg LW, Zuidema WC, et al. Encouraging psychological outcomes after altruistic donation to a stranger. American Journal of Transplantation. 2010;**10**(6):1445-1452

[27] Kaplan BS, Polise K. In defense of altruistic kidney donation by strangers. Pediatric Nephrology. 2000;**14**(6):518-522

[28] Spital A. Unconventional living kidney donors--attitudes and use among transplant centers. Transplantation. 1989;**48**(2):243-248

[29] Budiani-Saberi DA, Delmonico FL. Organ trafficking and transplant tourism: A commentary on the global realities. American Journal of Transplantation. 2008;**8**(5):925-929

[30] Ghods AJ. Renal transplantation in Iran. Nephrology, Dialysis, Transplantation. 2002;**17**(2):222-228

[31] Ghods AJ, Savaj S. Iranian model of paid and regulated living-unrelated kidney donation. Clinical Journal of the American Society of Nephrology. 2006;**1**(6):1136-1145

[32] Daar AS. The case for a regulated system of living kidney sales. Nature Clinical Practice. Nephrology. 2006;**2**(11):600-601

[33] Matas AJ. The case for living kidney sales: Rationale, objections and concerns. American Journal of Transplantation. 2004;**4**(12):2007-2017

[34] Matas AJ. Why we should develop a regulated system of kidney sales: A call for action! Clinical Journal of the American Society of Nephrology. 2006;**1**(6):1129-1132

Chapter 4

Organ Donation: Demand and Supply

Nadeem Ahmad Khan and Taqi Taufique Khan

Abstract

With its widening indications, the need for organ transplantation is growing globally. Currently, there is a crisis of organ shortage and a dire need to adopt ways and means to overcome it to save lives and improve the quality of life of patients with end-stage organ failure. In this regard, on the one hand, efforts should be made to eliminate the barriers to organ donation, such as people's ignorance about organ donation and ethical and religious concerns. On the other hand, strategies should be implemented to enhance organ donation, which in the case of deceased donors, include accelerating the donation process, instituting a policy of presumed or mandated consent, and utilizing extended criteria for donors. In the case of living donors, these include accepting the paired donation and removing disincentives to donation. Organ donation can also be boosted by allowing restricted compensation or reward. Using social media platforms to educate people, facilitate contacts, and match with unspecified donors is also worthwhile. In the future, xenotransplantation is also showing some promise.

Keywords: organ donation, donor organs, transplantation, living organ donation, desensitization techniques

1. Introduction

The availability of donor organs is a fundamental prerequisite for running a transplantation program. While the need for organ transplantation and its scope continues to expand, unfortunately, there continues to be a significant demand-supply gap in respect of potential donors, impeding the full exploitation of transplantation to save lives or improve the quality of life of patients with end-stage organ failure [1–3]. The problem can be traced back to myriad global causes, though some afflict particular countries due to their peculiar sociodemographic characteristics. Generally, lack of awareness, ethical concerns, religious dogma, and logistical problems are the major barriers to organ donation [4]. Overcoming them would require devising multifaceted strategies aiming at expanding all possible sources of donors. Living donations need particular emphasis since the pool of deceased donors is limited and cannot expand beyond a certain point due to inherited constraints [5, 6]. Furthermore, in addition to in-vogue strategies, some forward-thinking initiatives will be required for a substantial improvement in the situation.

1.1 Issues in organ donation

These may be universal or linked to the donor type. They broadly can be either deceased or living. The former is further classified as DBD (donation after brain death) or DCD (donation after cardiac death), while the latter is specified or unspecified [7]. The specified donors, in turn, can be directed (to a genetically related, emotionally related, or unrelated recipient) or undirected (through an exchange program); the unspecified donors are for anonymous recipients.

Some commonly encountered obstacles to organ donation are:

1.1.1 Awareness about organ donation

Even though transplantation has been around for many years, surprisingly most people in the general population, and also, in the medical community do not have adequate information about organ donation and transplantation [8, 9]. Even in developed societies, ignorance still reigns supreme, making it one of the most significant obstacles to organ donation [10].

This level of ignorance breeds skepticism toward the whole concept of transplantation. For instance, people might believe that professionals might be overly eager to remove donor organs to benefit potential recipients, even if this comes at the expense of the donors' interests—not knowing it is the donor or the donor's family who are the main stakeholders and have the final say in the matter [11]. These concerns can be alleviated only by educating people and informing them of every step of the organ donation process so they can make an informed decision about the donation [5, 12]. An independent donor advocacy team is also a step toward removing any misgivings regarding donor safety and rights [13]. All such measures can go a long way in ending the stigma associated with the practice of transplantation.

The dissemination of information regarding donation opportunities can significantly increase the proportion of potential donors [12, 14, 15]. For instance, Facebook's initiative to educate people about organ donation has led to a noticeable increase in the number of people in the United States who have signed up to become organ donors [16]. Another observation is that when people are provided with additional information about brain death, it makes them more willing to accept it, which speeds up the process of organ donation as a direct result [17].

1.1.2 Ethical issues

Organ donation may be hampered by several ethical issues which are directly linked to the process. Such concerns may arise when it comes to the following:

- Consent of donors
- Definition of death
- Nondirected living donation
- Donation of organs by patients of euthanasia
- Practice of rewarding or incentivizing organ donation.

- Online campaigns to encourage organ donation
- Xenotransplantation-related issues, such as animal rights, human dignity, risk of stem-cell technology, and genetic editing.

1.1.3 Consenting to organ donation

Consent that satisfies ethical standards should, in theory, be given of one's own free will and motivated solely by altruism; it should never be given in response to any form of pressure or coercion, nor should it be persuaded by the promise of monetary gain. However, in actual practice, it is difficult to determine objectively to what extent these standards are or could be followed [18]. As a consequence of this, there will always be some degree of uncertainty present. This inescapable shortfall in the process negatively impacts the populace's perception of transplantation as a whole.

Major ethical concerns about organ donation by living-related donors focus on the possibility of undue influence and emotional pressure and coercion by the recipients or their relatives to the point where the donor may be harmed.

Giving one's consent in the event of donation after death can take many different forms, but none is immune to ethical questions. In the *opt-in* option, those eligible to donate their organs do so voluntarily in life so that their organs can be harvested after they pass away. In some countries, the family is still allowed to decline the donation—referred to as the "soft option," as opposed to the "hard option," in which the family does not have this choice [19]. In the *opt-ou*t system, consent is treated as a default option, and if there is no declaration to the contrary from the deceased person, the consent is presumed to have been given. Though the opt-out option has been adopted by many countries, the ethical question of whether or not presumed consent accurately reflects the wishes of the deceased and violates donor autonomy continues to be debated [20]. Furthermore, it creates an even greater potential for abuse of power by medical professionals [21]. Not the least, there is yet no clear evidence that the opt-out option has increased the donation rate to any extent [21, 22].

A modification to the opt-out is the *mandated consent*, which means that all adults eligible for organ donation must register their intention to donate or not during life [22]. In this way, the wishes of the deceased individual would be honored posthumously regardless of the position held by the family. However, ethical concerns remain regarding individuals who either do not register or whose families are denied access to their medical records [23].

Organ conscription is a relatively new concept that refers to harvesting all healthy organs after death for transplantation regardless of the recipient's consent [24].

Living donors are free of the above issues but pose physical, psychological, and social challenges and there is always an element of doubt about their interpersonal relations and the motive behind the donation [6, 8].

1.1.4 Controversies about brain death

Even though death, as determined by neurological criteria, has been a legal definition of death for quite some time, the legitimacy of brain death determination has been called into question ever since its initial implementation, and various clinical scenarios continue to appear which give rise to medical, legal, and ethical controversies [25]. Furthermore, the inconsistencies within personal and institutional practices in establishing brain death, combined with the differences in legislation in various countries, raise the possibility of error in the diagnosis, thus adding to public discontentment [4, 26].

On the other hand, many religious and cultural communities still recognize death based on circulatory criteria, that is, irreversible cessation of heartbeat, and not neurological criteria [27]. Nevertheless, the issue is under continuing debate in these circles [28].

1.1.5 Non-directed living donation

There is an ongoing debate on the question of whether or not the practice of non-directed living donation is ethically justifiable [7, 29]. It is because it leaves a lacuna for illicit financial dealings or any other illegitimate arrangement between the donor and recipient [18].

1.1.6 Organ donation by euthanasia patients

Donating organs after a person has committed suicide with assistance is a relatively new concept that has raised new ethical questions [30]. Further, patients in this situation have the option of giving their permission to have their organs removed from their bodies while they are still alive. Not only does this remove concerns about obtaining consent after death, but it also makes it possible to retrieve organs while they are still healthy [31]. However, the possibility of pressuring potential donors into deciding on assisted suicide earlier than they otherwise would have is an ethical dilemma that needs to be solved for this practice to be considered morally acceptable [30, 31].

1.1.7 Rewards and incentives for organ donation

Notwithstanding its tremendous potential to boost organ donation, it is considered unethical to commercialize human organs or to make them as items of exchange or trade because the use of human body as an object violates an individual's dignity. Therefore, in the majority of nations, organ donation is only possible from "altruistic" donors; this means that no monetary or other forms of material value can be exchanged for a donor organ [29]. However, after much debate and exchange of arguments for and against paying donors, most authorities now agree that the expenses incurred by the donor in going through the process of organ donation can be reimbursed as these could be substantial [5, 12]. However, such payments should not be to the extent to become a financial incentive or disincentive to becoming a donor. Some other permissible ways of compensation could be exemptions from paying taxes, giving registered donors allocation priority, covering funeral costs, and making payments for unforeseen expanses [12, 32, 33].

1.1.8 Online platforms for organ donors

Finding living kidney organ donors online is made possible in the United States and the United Kingdom by the availability of online platforms containing registered altruistic living donors [12]. Though the facility dramatically simplifies the living donation process and lessens the strain on the waiting lists, it is shrouded in controversy since it is impossible to conclusively rule out the possibility of rewarding donations despite the undertakings made by the stakeholders to the contrary [34].

1.1.9 Religious issues

There is not a single religion in the world that is entirely against organ donation as all belief systems share common values of altruism, reverence for the sacredness of the human body, and respect for human dignity. Therefore, the majority accept organ donation as long as there is the donor's consent, no significant risks are involved, and actual deaths are verified in the case of deceased donors [27].

However, some Muslim jurists, Christian scholars, and Jewish rabbis are against it, particularly concerning deceased donors, primarily because of the debates surrounding the concept of what constitutes death [35]. Even though a minority holds it, this viewpoint may significantly influence organ donation in predominately religious communities [36].

In order to counter the fallouts of such negative religious trends, it is of the utmost importance to actively engage religious leaders and organizations in the drive for organ donation [27]. For instance, a person of faith might be included right at the beginning during the family counseling process after a donor has been declared brain dead.

1.1.10 Logistic issues

Setting up a deceased donor program on a national level is administratively quite demanding. In addition to political will and extensive infrastructure, there is also a need for a committed organization with dedicated leadership, a trained human source, and networking with intensive care units (ICUs). It is, therefore, quite understandable that while the developed countries have well-established deceased donor programs, patients in developing and undeveloped countries, except a few, are deprived of this important donor source [37, 38].

1.2 Developments in Prevailing practices

Deceased donors, which primarily involve donation after brain death (DBD), continue to be the primary sources of donor organs in countries where the program has been established on a national level. Donations after circulatory death (DCD) supplement the deceased donor source but at the cost of inferior outcomes [3, 39]. Despite their inclusion, however, the number of deceased donors has not increased enough to meet the demand; in fact it has reached a plateau in most countries [6].

1.2.1 Improving the efficiency of the deceased donor program

By identifying potential donors early in intensive care units, the necessary medical and legal procedures, including family counseling, can be completed early, thereby protecting the organs from the pathophysiological changes in the body that come with brain death [24]. Appropriate training and persuasion of the ICU staff and transplant coordinators can also help in timely referrals and their conversion to actual donors [31].

Including expanded-criteria-donors (ECD) could also help increase the deceased donor pool [22]. Similarly, drug intoxication as the cause of death should no longer be considered a contraindication to organ donation, and kidney transplants from HIV-positive donors to HIV-positive recipients are also permissible [40].

1.2.2 Improvements in living donation

In the case of living-donors, their scope can also be increased by expanding their eligibility criteria. For instance, if otherwise fit, people aged up to 70 or having obesity or vascular malformation can also be accepted as donors [5, 41]. Living-unrelated donors are another area that deserves greater attention. Despite not sharing a genetic connection with the recipient, the graft outcome is similar to that obtained from living-related donors [42]. These donors might have emotional ties with the recipients or be strangers, getting motivated for donation by knowing the potential recipient's need through an intermediary person, the media, or public solicitation. Such a donation may be directed or undirected in exchange for priority of donor's family member listed for the deceased donor [3].

The paired donor exchange in which two donors exchange kidneys among their respective recipients because of their blood or tissue incompatibility with the original donor is yet another way of increasing the living donor donation rate [43]. In practical terms, the exchange works by assisting donor/patient pairs with incompatible blood types to find another donor/patient pair with whom they are compatible with exchanging kidneys. There are currently paired kidney programs operating in the United Kingdom (UK), a few other European countries, and as a pilot project in the United States [3].

Domino transplantation provides yet another source of donor organs [44]. In this method, one donor makes a contribution to the recipient of an incompatible couple. The second donor, known as the domino-donor, then makes a contribution to either another couple or the waiting list. In contrast to kidney-exchange donation, which necessitates the mutual compatibility of both the recipient and donor couples, domino-paired donation does not require such compatibility between the parties. Another form of domino-donation involves donating the kidney or liver of an individual who has already received a transplant to another person on a waiting list for one of those organs.

1.3 New approaches

As a result of the ongoing disparity between organ supply and demand, Investigations are being conducted into various alternative options, such as xenotransplantation and artificial organs which can help in reducing the burden of potential recipients. For example, artificial extracorporeal liver support devices capable of performing hemodialysis, therapeutic plasma exchange (TPE), and albumin dialysis have been developed in recent years. TPE has been shown to improve patients' chances of surviving acute liver failure in clinical trials, and these trials show that the devices are safe and well tolerated by patients [45]. In addition, a total artificial heart (TAH), also known as mechanical circulatory support that restores total pulmonary and systemic flow, is an alternative option for people currently waiting for a donor's heart [46]. Similarly, wearable artificial kidneys are also under clinical trials presently [47].

The practice of xenotransplantation, also known as the transplantation of pig organs into humans, has been brought one step closer to becoming a reality because of recent developments in techniques of gene editing which allow breeding pigs free of xenoantigens and porcine endogenous retroviruses—the two main causes of failure of previous attempts in this direction [48].

However, even though these alternative methods hold promise, they present several challenges and concerns about the source of organs, animal rights, human dignity, and potential organ transplant potential carcinogenicity of stem-cell research, as well as improperly employing genetic techniques. Thus, research in this direction requires tight regulation.

2. Conclusion

Organ donation is a multifaceted field that, in addition to medical and scientific concerns, involves the interaction of social, religious, ethical, and legal domains. Therefore, it is necessary to take a multipronged approach to meet the ever-increasing demand of patients who are candidates for organ transplantation. However, checks and balances should always be in place to ensure that donors are safe and their rights are protected.

Author details

Nadeem Ahmad Khan* and Taqi Taufique Khan
Department of Kidney Transplantation, Rehman Medical Institute, Peshawar, Pakistan

*Address all correspondence to: n_ahmad_2000@yahoo.co.uk

References

[1] OPTN data. 2022 Available from: https://optn.transplant.hrs.gov/data

[2] Available from: https://www.organdonor.gov

[3] Wynn JJ, Alexander CE. Increasing organ donation and transplantation: The U.S. experience over the past decade. Transplant International. 2011;**24**:324-332

[4] Da Silva IRF, Frontera JA. Worldwide barriers to organ donation. JAMA Neurology. 2015;**72**:112-118

[5] Saidi RF, Hejazii Kenari SK. Challenges of organ shortage for transplantation: Solutions and opportunities. International Journal of Organ Transplantation Medicine. 2014;**5**:87-96

[6] Lennerling A, Lovén C, Dor FJ, Ambagtsheer F, Duerinckx N, Frunza M, et al. Living organ donation practices in Europe – Results from an online survey. Transplant International. 2013;**26**:145-153

[7] Dor FJMF, Massey EK, Frunza M, et al. New classification of ELPAT for living organ donation. Transplantation. 2011;**91**(9):935-938

[8] Irving MJ, Tong A, Jan S, Cass A, Rose J, Chadban S, et al. Factors that influence the decision to be an organ donor: A systematic review of the qualitative literature. Nephrology Dialysis Transplantation. 2011;**27**:2526-2533

[9] Atamañuk AN, Ortiz Fragola JP, Giorgi M, Berreta J, Lapresa S, Ahuad-Guerrero A, et al. Medical students' attitude toward organ donation: Understanding reasons for refusal in order to increase transplantation rates. Transplantation Proceedings. 2018;**50**:2976-2980

[10] Horton RL, Horton PJ. Knowledge regarding organ donation: Identifying and over- coming barriers to organ donation. Social Science & Medicine. 1990;**31**:791-800

[11] Newton JD. How does the general public view posthumous organ donation? A meta-synthesisof the qualitative literature. BMC Public Health. 2011;**11**:791

[12] Abouna GM. Organ shortage crisis: Problems and possible solutions. Transplantation Proceedings. 2008;**40**:34-38

[13] Robbins CK. The independent living donor advocate: An essential role for living kidney donation. Nephrology Nursing Journal. 2014;**41**(6):569-573

[14] Mucsi I, Novak M, Toews D, Waterman A. Explore Transplant Ontario: adapting the explore transplant education program to facilitate informed decision making about kidney transplantation. Canadian Journal of Kidney Health and Disease. 2018;**24**:5

[15] Waterman AD, Rodrigue JR. Transplant and organ donation education: What matters? Progress in Transplantation. 2009;**19**:7-8

[16] Cameron AM, Massie AB, Alexander CE, Stewart B, Montgomery RA, Benavides N, et al. Social media and organ donor registration: The Facebook effect. American Journal of Transplantation. 2013;**13**:2059-2065

[17] Cohen B, Wight C. A European perspective on organ procurement: Breaking down the barriers to organ donation. Transplantation. 1999;**68**:985-990

[18] Epstein M. Danovitch G is altruistic-directed living unrelated organ donation a legal fiction? Nephrology Dialysis Transplantation. 2009;**24**(2):357-360

[19] Shepherd L, O'Carroll RE, Ferguson E. An international comparison of deceased and living organdonation/ transplant rates in opt-in andopt-out systems: A panel study. BMC Medicine. 2014;**12**:131

[20] Prabhu PK. Is presumed consent an ethically acceptable way of obtaining organs for transplant? Journal of Intensive Care. 2019;**20**(2):92-97

[21] Orentlicher D. Presumed consent to organ donation: its rise and fall in the United States. Rutgers Law Review. 2008;**61**:295-331

[22] Etheredge HR. Assessing Global Organ Donation Policies: Opt-In vs Opt-Out Risk Manag Healthc Policy. 2021;**14**:1985-1998

[23] Cotter H. Increasing consent for organ donation: Mandated choice, individual au- tonomy, and informed consent. Health Matrix. 2011;**21**:599

[24] Spital A. Conscription of cadaveric organs for transplantation: A stimulating idea whose time has not yet come. Cambridge Quarterly of Healthcare Ethics. 2005;**14**:107-112

[25] Youn TS, Greer DM. Brain death and Management of a Potential Organ Donor in the intensive care unit. Critical Care Clinics. 2014;**30**:813-831

[26] Lewis A, Lord AS, Czeisler BM, Caplan A. Public education and misinformation on brain death in mainstream media. Clinical Transplantation. 2016;**30**:1082-1089

[27] Jones DA. Loss of faith in brain death: Catholic controversy over the determination of death by neurological criteria. Clinical Ethics. 2012;**7**:133-141

[28] Randhawa G, Brocklehurst A, Pateman R, Kinsella S, Parry V. Religion and organ donation: The views of UK faith leaders. Journal of Religion and Health. 2012;**51**:743-751

[29] Steinberg D. The allocation of organs donated by altruistic strangers. Annals of Internal Medicine. 2006;**145**:197-203

[30] Somerville M. Does it matter how we die? Ethical and legal issues raised by combining euthanasia and organ transplantation. The Linacre Quarterly. 2019;**86**:359-365

[31] Philpot SJ. Organ donation after circulatory death following voluntary assisted dying: Practicaland ethical considerations for Victoria. Critical Care and Resuscitation. 2018;**20**:254

[32] Levy M. State incentives to promote organ donation: Honoring the principles of reciprocity and solidarity inherent in the gift relationship. Journal of Law and the Biosciences. 2018;**5**:398-435

[33] Matas AJ, Satel S, Munn S, Richards JR, Tan-Alora A, et al. Incentives for organ donation: Proposed standards for an internationally acceptable system. American Journal of Transplantation. 2012;**12**:306-312 9

[34] Limb M. Organ matching website says it will operate within the law. BMJ. 2012;**345**:e6030

[35] Oliver M, Ahmed A, Woywodt A. Donating in good faith or getting into

trouble re- ligion and organ donation revisited. World Journal of Transplantation. 2012;**2**:69

[36] Fortin MCW-JB. Should we perform kidney transplants on foreign nationals? Journal of Medical Ethics. 2014;**40**:821-826

[37] Silva D, Hareendra E, Godakandage MHP, et al. Deceased donor organ donation in a developing country; an early experience in a tertiary Care Center in Sri Lanka. Transplantation. 2017;**101**:S52

[38] Abraham G, Vijayan M, Gopalakrishnan N, et al. State of deceased donor transplantation in India: A model for developing countries around the world. World Journal of Transplantation. 2016;**6**(2):331-335

[39] Blackstock MJ, Ray DC. Organ donation after circulatory death: An update. European Journal of Emergency Medicine. 2014;**21**:324-329

[40] Botha J, Fabian J, Etheredge H, Conradie F, Tiemessen CT. HIV and solid organ trans- plantation: Where are we now. Current HIV/AIDS Reports. 2019;**16**:404-413

[41] Ahmadi AR, Lafranca JA, Claessens LA, Imamdi RMS, Ijzermans JNM, Betjes MGH, et al. Shifting paradigms in eligibility criteria for live kidney donation: A systematic review. Kidney International. 2015;**87**:31-45

[42] Matoka MC, Switzer G. Nondirected living donation: A survey of current trends and practices. Transplantation. 2005;**79**:515-519

[43] RRatner LE, Rana A, Ratner ER, et al. The altruistic Unbalanced paired kidney exchange: Proof of concept and survey of potential donor and recipient attitude. Transplantation. 2010;**89**(1):15-22

[44] Roodnat JI, Zuidema W, van de Wetering J, et al. Altruistic donor triggered domino-paired kidney donation for unsuccessful couples from the kidney-exchange program. American Journal of Transplantation. 2010;**10**:821

[45] Larsen FS. Artificial liver support in acute and acute-on-chronic liver failure. Current Opinion in Critical Care. 2019;**25**:187-191

[46] Copeland JG, Arabia FA, Tsau PH, Nolan PE, McClellan D, Smith RG, et al. Total artificial hearts: Bridge to transplantation. Cardiology Clinics. 2003;**21**(1):101-113

[47] Huff C. How artificial kidneys and miniaturized dialysis could save millions of lives. Nature. 2020;**579**(7798):186-188

[48] Loike JD, Kadish A. Ethical rejections of xenotransplantation? The potential and challenges of using human-pig chimeras to create organs for transplantation. EMBO Reports. 2018;**19**(8):1-4

Chapter 5

Nauseous Nexus between the Organ Industry and the Risks of Illegal Organ Harvesting

Karen R.V. Francis-Cummings

Abstract

Organ transplantation saves lives and provides the best alternative for patients at the end-stage of their illness. Interestingly in some jurisdictions, a person who knowingly buys or sell organs for transplantation, could be penalized. However, there continues to be a lucrative global trade and a booming business in human organs as some companies prefer to remain as a private entity rather than undergo increase scrutiny by outside financiers. The common belief is that public health should be made to prevail over private wealth. Therefore, the troubling query is, why some health institutions that conduct organ and tissue transplantation are less transparent, and their work and processes shrouded in secrecy. The vulnerable, voiceless, and marginalized of society are more at risk with illegal organ harvesting activities. Donors' rights are violated as they benefit little economically, and the lack of donor information could result in serious health and social risks. Law enforcement officers struggle to offer the relevant intelligence for swift action by policy decision -makers. This chapter gives attention to and increase awareness among researchers and community activists that this special gift of organ donation appropriately scheduled should be of a high quality and improve the lives of persons terminally ill.

Keywords: illegal organ harvesting/trafficking, organ donation, organ transplantation, risks of illegal organ harvesting, ethics, organ transplantation and law

1. Introduction

It is indisputable that Organ transplantation has saved lives and has provided the best alternative for patients who are at terminal stages of their illnesses and who would have experienced end - stage organ failure. Evidently this phenomenon is a medical miracle and milestone. It is part of the gripping advances in health in this twenty-first century in multi-ethnic societies and in populations with diverse cultures. However, this medical breakthrough abounds with complexities. The wide gap between organ supply and organ demand gives rise to prolong waiting times to receive organs as well as the increasing mortality among several vulnerable persons on waiting lists. This is the main contributing factors to this challenge. Additionally, organ donation remains an extremely sensitive and topical issue in extremely religious societies. In those societies the emphasis continues to be placed more on the body of deceased persons [1]. This is because there is the perception that there are several factors that mitigate a potential donor from consenting to the donation of an organ or tissue for transplantation during life or after death.

According to Ali et al. [2], the issues raised would include the lack of information, misinformation, and disinformation concerning the donation of an organ, suspicion of a healthcare system, the attitudes and views of family members and religious leaders, and a clear ruling and interpretation of the rulings of the clergy. Therefore, with such a mindset, for candidates waiting for transplantation owing to their irreversible medical conditions, the possibility of a delay in waiting time and unequal access of organ donation could be further compromised.

The sources of organs for transplantation include living donor (related and nonrelated), cadaveric donor, and brain-dead patients [3]. It is necessary to further distinguish the four categories: 1) Living Related Organ Donation "blood or emotional" which is a directed donation to a loved one [3, 4]; 2) Altruistic Organ Donation: non-directed donation, in which the donor gives an organ to the general pool to be transplanted into the recipient at the top of the waiting list [3, 4]; 3) Living Non-Related Organ Donation: directed donation to a stranger, whereby donors choose to give to a specific person with whom they have no prior emotional connection [3]; and 4) Cross donation where a living donor wants to donate to his blood or emotional relative an organ but blood groups does not match and there is a complete mismatch or cross matching is positive [3, 4].

According to Saleh [5], the kidneys are the most transplanted organ. The author further stated that in 2011, 11, 835 deceased -donor kidney transplants and 5, 772 living -donor transplants had occurred. [6] also reported that in the year 2021, there was more organ transplants ever in a single year and there was an eight percent increase in kidney transplant. Kidney transplant had moved from 22, 817 in 2020 to 24, 670 in 2021.

World Health Organization (WHO) [7] has reported that noncommunicable diseases (NCDs) is responsible for the deaths of 41 million people annually and 71 percent of the deaths globally. According to WHO [7], each year, 15 million people die from a NCD between the ages of 30 and 69 years, while 85 percent of these "premature" deaths occur in low- and middle-income countries accounting for seventy-seven percent of all NCD deaths. The increase of morbidity and mortality for NCDs has been attributed to the modifiable behaviors including unhealthy diets and a lack of physical activity, leading to severe hypertension and diabetes. According to WHO [8], globally, 422 million people live with diabetes whereas 62 million people in the Americas live with Diabetes Mellitus (DM) type II. WHO [8] further reported that Diabetes accounts for 244,084 deaths annually and in addition, 1.5 million cases of diabetes globally are directly attributed to diabetes each year thus accounting for 45 percent of new cases of chronic kidney disease diagnosed annually. Chen [9] has reported that over the past three decades, diabetes has become one of the most important public health challenges to all nations as the number of people with diabetes mellitus has more than doubled globally. In addition, medical expenditures have been 2.3 times higher than what expenditures would be in the absence of diabetes. According to American Diabetes Association [10], the indirect costs would include an increase in absenteeism ($3.3 billion) and reduced productivity while at work ($26.9 billion) for the employed population, reduced productivity for those not in the labor force ($2.3 billion), inability to work because of disease-related disability ($37.5 billion), and lost productivity due to 277,000 premature deaths attributed to diabetes ($19.9 billion). Cantrovich [11] had reported that shortage of organs could be a social, psychological, ethical, moral, and political problem, causing unjustifiable damage to public health.

2. Trends in illegal harvesting and benefits from the lucrative business

Surgical procedures like transplant of an organ would be morally acceptable with the consent of the donor and without excessive risks for the waiting patient. And that this noble act of organ donation must occur after death, where the real death of the donor must be fully ascertained. Interestingly, in Nigeria, organ trafficking is considered or rather is divided into three categories, namely firstly) the traffickers who would trick the victims into surrendering his organ at no cost; secondly, the "con -artist" who would convince gullible victims into selling their organs but somehow end up not paying them the agreed sum or not at all; and thirdly, this category would include the doctors who would treat patients for ailment that are non -existent and by extension remove the organs without the victims knowledge [12].

According to Cerón et al. [13], organ harvesting occurs to facilitate healthy and viable organs, primarily kidneys, to the wealthier individuals who require a transplant option and are unable to get it through more legal means and which may include the family and close friends. Cerón et al. [13] further reported that organs are usually either be sold or stolen from the "donor" owing to the economic supply and demand of the organ, and later are transferred to the purchaser for transplantation. Kar and Spanjers [14] noted that the illegal organ donation industry would generate $US840 million to 1.7 billion dollars annually. The common organs include kidney $US 8 million, liver $US 3 million, heart $ US700,000, lung $ US 500,000 and the pancreas $US 200, 000. The location of transplantation would have taken place in Asia, including countries like China, Kosovo, and Singapore, in South Africa, and in the United States of America and in Peru, South America. The Author reported that there has been gross disparity between the vendors and the recipients' fees, as the vendors receive less than 10 percent of the recipient's payment while the "middlemen" usually receive the lion's share of the sum.

According to Tao [15], 10 percent of the 63,000 kidneys transplanted worldwide each year from living donors have been bought illegally. Tao [15] further reported that with kidney continuing to top the list of organ illegal trade with at least two hourly and that being 75 percent of the global illegal trade in organs. In 2014, 8000 illegal kidney transplants were performed although the prices varied according to nationality and location [14]. Kar & Spanjers [14] reported that while the price for a kidney transplant had cost $30,000, countries like Israel and Indonesia the cost of a kidney transplant had been $25, 000 and $23, 000 respectively; in Japan the cost was $16, 000, while there was a $4, 000 difference in China (12,000) for the said organ while for a similar organ in Peru was $12,000. According to Sharif et al. [16], the unethical nature of using organs from executed prisoners, due to its limitations on voluntary and informed consent in China has been unanimously stated in literature. Though this practice has been frowned and denounced by international declarations including the Nuremberg Code, the Helsinki Declaration, the Belmont report, Amnesty International, the World Health Organization, the World Medical Association (WMA), and of recent by the Declaration of Istanbul, but incarcerated inmates condemned to death may still not be in the position to make an autonomous and informed consent for organ donation in China [16].

According to Bruckmuller [17], the first official investigated case of illegal organ sale and trafficking was recorded in Bombay, India in 1993, however, the doctor in charge was only captured in 2008. Similarly, in the United States, after ten years, a physician- in -charge was eventually prosecuted for heading an illegal organ transplant ring. The Author further stressed that there have been other cases documented throughout the world owing to a well strategic operations with multiple individuals such as middlemen who constantly move various organ parts within the process of the transaction. In recent times, the Indian authorities claimed to have broken up a ring involving doctors, nurses, paramedics, and hospitals that had performed 500 illegal transplants of organs to rich Indians and foreigners. Most of the donors were poor laborers who were paid up to $2500 for a kidney.

World Health Organization [8] reported that in 2021, the authorities in India had broken up a ring involving doctors, nurses, paramedics, and hospitals that had performed 500 illegal transplants of organs to rich Indians and foreigners. Most of the donors were poor laborers who were paid up to $2500 for a kidney. Some were forced to give up organs at gunpoint. Bruckmuller [17] noted that the shortage of needed organs could lead to the patient's willingness to pay high sums of money for body parts, especially organs. According to Bruckmuller [17], the Criminal organizations which have occurred in cooperation with staff members of the healthcare sector are very lucrative business with the trade of body parts, especially with the offense on human trafficking for organ (cells and tissue) removal.

3. What are the potential risks of illegal organ trafficking

Bos [18] has reported that the at-risk population namely the organ suppliers and victims can be classified into eight categories. These categories include but are not limited to 1) persons who have come from the less developed countries where the majority of persons are below the poverty line; 2) persons with the status of an immigrant or of a refugee; 3) persons who are very vulnerable; 4) persons who would have lacked knowledge in medical sciences and are unaware of what it means to have the removal of a kidney; 5) the victims are usually uneducated and illiterate; 6) the victims are usually young males within the 18 to 30 age group; 7) persons that could be easily coerced and deceived into obtaining the organ and 8) the victims who usually come from counties of origin where there is either a lack of a proper functioning legislative system that forbids such practice or countries which are unable to prosecute individuals owing to a high level of corruption. According to Bos [18], these victims and donors have been left to care for themselves following the removal of their organs and the final payments have been made. The Author further stated that the local recruiters are usually prevented from lodging complaints to the authorities owing to the lack of knowledge and awareness as to the importance of removing an organ and the punishment that might be available. Apart for the donor's rights being violated most of the times, there has been limited economic benefits that are seen with the suppliers.

Illegal organ harvesting has been associated with complaints of asthenia, pain and health complications, the deterioration of the victim's health usually because of inadequate post-operative care, and job loss [18]. Interestingly and frequently, it has been difficult to trace the whereabouts of the organ suppliers. When considering the potential risks of illegal organ trafficking, attention must also be paid to the health risks of the recipients. Bos [18] has noted that there could be serious health and social risks for the persons who are selling the organs as they are unable to give much clarity to the recipients of the commercial transplants. The Author further stated that when a comparison is made between the developed countries like the United States of America, the United Kingdom, Canada, Australia and Turkey and other less developed countries dealing with organ transplantation, there have been better outcomes from the type of transplant received from the developed when compared to the developing countries. There have been less surgical complications, post-operation hernia, infections from the wound or donor derived, less instances of infectious and sexually transmitted diseases, acute myocardial infarction, steroid diabetes, and inferior graft have been reported from recipients from the developed countries [19]. However, when compared to the developing countries, there were less patient survival and lack of data and information relating to donor information. According to UNODC [19], the grave effects of the illegal organ trade have been the increase in children mortality rate worldwide. The giving of impulsive donation by non-compensated donors without written consent and a stated waiting period. The Author further noted that the increasing network of criminality, especially the kidnapping of children and teenagers, who are murdered, and their organs harvested have been striking.

4. Challenges to enforcement

Despite stringent efforts by the European parliament and the United Nations making declaration and resolutions to "fight "against the trafficking of organs and putting rigorous measures in place to punish health care providers who condone and participate in the system of illegal trafficking of organs, the challenge to enforce appropriate laws to stop this illegal practice continues. According to Francis and Francis [20], the International Criminal Court (ICC) is not constructed to address transboundary crimes. However, the need to prosecute the offender and to address illegal organ trafficking is not without serious challenges, especially among states that are big on tourism. According to Adido [21], because of the illegal nature of the activities that are involved in the organ transplant tourism which includes secrecy under which some of the illegal activities are undertaken. With corrupt practices alleged to be occurring among the organ brokers, the enforcement officers, and regulatory bodies are all experiencing formidable challenges to enforcing appropriate laws. Ambagtsheer [22] reported that judges and prosecutors in Kosovo had refused to issue valid orders for a search and arrest on several individuals who were high members of the judiciary and who had refused to testify citing the case that they were off duty and that they were not paid for their duties after hours. However, the Author further noted that local factors such as poverty, corruption, poor regulation, weak enforcement methods, the inadequate local laws and cultural practices all help to mitigate the curtailing of this topical issue.

According to Ambagtsheer [22], the payment for organs should be banned because of the possible unfair treatment of the poor and vulnerable and even those persons who undermine altruistic donation of the organs. It has also been noted that the absence of measures of accountability and the inability of the lawmakers to identify the agencies that would be able to implement such laws could compromise any developing institutional structure and provide legal uncertainty [22]. Cerón et al. [13] reported that the main challenge to the enforcement of laws to illegal organ trafficking would be threat of the lack of resources, ineffectiveness of law enforcement, animosities between communities and the government, organs for donation through confidentiality agreements under the guise of law, and organ seizures from some category of medical practitioners. However, as there remains lucrative incentives for both the purchase and sales of organs in both affluent and impoverished areas of the world, efforts of prevention would be simply prescriptive but lack a regime of enforcement [20].

5. Recommendations

Untiring efforts have been made by countries in the Caribbean, Asia, and in the Metropolitan to stem the tide of illegal organ harvesting. In fact, several principles have been established and advanced from the Asian Task force on Organ Trafficking to the Declaration of Istanbul 2018 to strengthen lack of donation records, the inadequate regulation for donation of deceased donors, and limited human resources with the correct expertise has contributed to the inequitable access to organ transplants and organ trafficking [23]. According to WHO [8], health is not just the absence of disease but that there must be the consideration of the total well-being of the individual: Family physicians and primary care physicians (PCPs) should play a key role in health promotion and in disease prevention.

According to Kao [24], the physicians should be compelled to act in a way that promotes equity and enhances the chances of all persons to live a healthy life especially when considering the social determinants of health. The Author further stated that physicians should guard against the "Pittsburg protocol" of practicing the retrieval of organs for donation from non-heart- beating rather than from brain-dead donors. It behooves the family members to ask about donation before the life support is removed to prevent valuable time being lost, and the organs become unsuitable for transplantation.

The physician can be of great help to the patients by discussing the significance of organ donation. The importance of disseminating such information could benefit the patients in four reasons. Firstly, the PCPs would have an established relationship of trust with patients, being more aware of the patient's cultural and moral preferences and hence would be able to better tailor information and engage in shared decision making [25], Secondly, according to Thornton et al. [25], the ambulatory setting may be particularly well suited for discussions about organ donation because people under the age of 50, who comprise over a third of deceased organ donors, utilize ambulatory services at disproportionately high rates. Thirdly, PCPs have successfully engaged in difficult conversations about end-of-life care that have increased the number of patients who completed in advance [26]; and fourth and finally, for patients, designating donor status would allow them to preserve their autonomy, give them piece of mind, and permit them to feel confident that they have contributed to their end-of-life care and treatment by documenting and communicating their wishes in case situations arise in which they would be unable to do so ([27]; National Survey of Organ Donation Attitudes and Behaviors. Rockville, MD: [27]).

To decrease the risk of illegal organ harvesting and to bring a halt to this booming and lucrative industry, there must be the combined effort of government and non-government institutions to prevent such crimes, to protect the vulnerable and marginalized donors, and to prosecute the agencies or persons engaged in corrupt practices.

The recommendations for consideration include but not limited to the following suggestions:

6. Prevention

a. To increase the supply of organs donated through media which would guard against exploitation by donors who are willing and able to donate their organ [28].

b. To enhance the donor pool in well-resourced countries to meet their own needs and,

c. To upgrade facilities and standardize medical care [28].

7. Protection

a. To have regulated, standardized, and ethical system for organ procurement [28].

b. To have Presumed Consent Policies on Organ Trade- According to Bamgbose [12], presumed consent policies could curb organ trafficking while simultaneously, increase the numbers of legal organ donations globally, land thus lessening the need for organ tourism.

c. To have an opt-in and an opt -out policy system of organ donation as is seen in countries successfully implemented like Brazil, the United States of America, and several European Nations where an individual may decide to donate his/her organ while still living. In addition, Bamgbose [12], also reported that an opt-out organ donation policy system would be needed as such policy would suggest that organ donation is done after death.

d. To have accountability measures with sanctions attached should be made which will make doctors liable if found associated in illegal organ transplantation.

e. To create awareness in the physicians and the public by ensuring that there is integrity in the pursuit of self-sufficiency [28],

f. To enforce legislation for transplantation- meaning that regulations, legislations, and agencies should be set up and put in place, adequately equipped with appropriate measures and sanctions to quell this disturbance of organ trade which is rising globally at a phenomenal pace Bamgbose [12].

g. To approve systems that will foster accountability, safety in surgical practices, employ vendor registries, provide donors with lifetime care, and include benefits or compensations, especially for volunteer donors as a means of appreciating and encouraging legal organ donation, whilst also reducing black market operations Bamgbose [12].

h. To adopt creative approaches by utilizing technological advancement set up to help expose misconducts and aid whistle blowing. Examples of these methods include: —Tor|| which is an anonymity network used globally by whistleblowers; Securedrop|| and —Global Leaks|| which have been adopted to enhance secure whistle blowing; and Open Board|| which is another security service used in whistle blowing internationally [12]. Whistle Blowing policy has taken several forms such as Internal, External, Third Party, Private Sector, and Public Sector; however, Internal Whistle Blowing is considered a good type to mitigating corruption and enhancing sustainable development as in Nigeria [12]

8. Prosecution

Another recommendation to assist in the prohibition of the illegal harvesting of Human Organ is to be able to prosecute the culprits. According to Gawronska et al. [29], there are two main conditions rather indications where prosecution should be meted out, namely, 1) if there was no consent to remove the human organ from a living donor and 2) if there were monetary benefits included in the arrangement without violating the principle of ne bis in idem as developed by the European Court of Human Rights (ECHR) and the Court of Justice of the European Union (CJEU).

However, Gawronska et al. [29] further reported that members of the judiciary and law enforcement should receive the proper training. The Author noted that there could be double prosecution of illicit organ removal as organ trafficking and the possibility to prosecute illicit organ removal under the human trafficking and organ trafficking frameworks, hence awareness must be raised of this overlap to avoid double prosecution and punishment. Gawronska et al. [29] noted that there could be a case, though, hypothetically, where the physician to whom a patient is transferred, proceeds to remove an organ in exchange for money. According to Gawronska et al. [29], such a case could involve not only a single act, but a plurality of acts: on the one hand, 'taking control over the victim' (which constitutes human trafficking within the meaning of Article 433quinquies, §1, of the Criminal Code) and, on the other, 'illicit organ removal' (penalized under Article 433novies/2 of the Criminal Code). Thus, there is therefore the possibility of a criminal court judge ruling that these punishable acts are interrelated through a common intention, objective, and execution and that they should therefore still be regarded as a single act [29].

Finally, to be able to prosecute effectively and to have successful organ trafficking case outcomes, there must be trained medical and forensic experts to assist with such investigation and to establish national reporting codes for identifying and disclosures of trafficking networks [30] Insurance companies must not support illegal practices [31]; a transparency of transplantation practice that is accountable to health authorities should be in place; and proper bilateral agreements should be established to permit the enhanced transfer of organs across countries and to address transboundary crimes [22].

9. Conclusion

In conclusion, this topical issue of Illegal Organ Harvesting continues to leave a destructive medical footprint owing to the exploitation of the poor and vulnerable in the low-income countries with serious health consequences while contributing significantly to the wealthy in the first world metropolitan. According to Zimik [32], because of poverty, ethnic conflicts, unemployment, gender inequality, inadequate legislation and law enforcement have enabled such trafficking of the illegal human organs to thrive. Importantly, the private sector and the financial industry have acted in concert and unknowingly have been a conduit for its facilitation [31]. The growing demand of human organs especially for the kidneys and livers by unscrupulous traffickers and the unhealthy lifestyles of some citizens have contributed to this global shortage of supply. It is the wish that where there are lax laws to encourage and support human organs being transferred via transboundary crossing or going directly to recipients in wealthier countries, be identified and fixed. The training of anti-money laundering professionals and law enforcement agents to detect related financial activity is imperative. In addition, epidemiological data and global transparency should be obtainable and visible to assist the living donors and recipients manage their long-term health, psychological and socio-economic consequences.

With the engagement of the right public-private partnerships, the meticulous international efforts of all stakeholders to identify illegal transplant activities, to investigate and disrupt and prosecute trafficking networks, I am optimistic that this age-old illegal and unlawful practice and booming business could be reduced significantly if not abolished. According to Okere & Emedolu [33], the Immanuel Kant's End formulation which elucidates that man should not be used to satisfy or serve another end as he would make the former a means to the latter as man's creative body is already an end this.

Acknowledgements

The Author is grateful to an anonymous reviewer for his assistance for thoughtful comments on an earlier draft of this chapter which helped to improve its quality. I also thank the funders for their monetary contributions toward this project.

Conflict of interest

"The author declares no conflict of interest."

Acronyms and abbreviations

AMA	American Diabetes Association
CJEU	Court of Justice of the European Union
DM	Diabetes Mellitus
ECHR	European Court of Human Rights
ICC	International Criminal Court
NCDS	Non-communicable diseases
PCP	Primary care physician
UNOC	United Nations on drugs and crime
UNODC	United Nations Office on Drug and Crime
UNOS	United Network for Organ Network
WMA	World Medical Association
WHO	World Health Organization

Author details

Karen R.V. Francis-Cummings
Guyana Parliament, Georgetown, Guyana

*Address all correspondence to: karen.cummings82@yahoo.com

References

[1] Sharp LA. Organ transplantation as a transformative experience: Anthropological insights into the restructuring of the self. Medical Anthropology Quarterly. 1995;**9**(3):357-389

[2] Ali A, Ahmed T, Ayub A, Dano S, Khalid M, El-Dassouki N, et al. Organ donation and transplant: The Islamic perspective. Clinical Transplantation. 2020;*34*(4):e13832

[3] Al-Bar MA, Chamsi-Pasha H. Organ transplantation. In: Contemporary Bioethics. Cham: Springer; 2015. pp. 209-225

[4] Lewis A, Koukoura A, Tsianos GI, Gargavanis AA, Nielsen AA, Vassiliadis E. Organ donation in the US and Europe: The supply vs demand imbalance. Transplantation Reviews. 2021;**35**(2):100585

[5] Saleh N. Top 6 single-organ transplants: More than 500,000 organ transplants have been done in the U.S. 2021. Available from: rywellhealth.com/common-single-organ-transplants-4082949

[6] United Network for Organ Sharing. Report. 2017. Available from: http://www.unos.org/

[7] World Health Organization. Non-Communicable Diseases: Key facts. 2021. Available from: https://www.who.int/news-room/fact-sheets/detail/noncommunicable-diseases

[8] World Health Organization. Diabetes: Key facts. 2022. Available from: https://www.who.int/news-room/fact-sheets/detail/diabetes

[9] Chen L, Magliano D, Zimmet P. The worldwide epidemiology of type 2 diabetes mellitus—Present and future perspectives. Nature Reviews. Endocrinology. 2012;**8**:228-236. DOI: 10.1038/nrendo.2011.183

[10] American Diabetes Association. Economic costs of diabetes in the US in 2017. Diabetes Care. 2018;**41**(5):917-928. DOI: 10.2337/dci18-0007

[11] Cantarovich F. The society, the barriers to organ donation and alternatives for a change. In: Organ Donation and Transplantation-Current Status and Future Challenges. London: IntechOpen; 2018. DOI: 10.5772/intechopen.73756. Available from: https://www.intechopen.com/chapters59201

[12] Bamgbose O. Human Organ Trade: Trending Issues and the Relationship to Access to Justice. Nigeria: University of Ibadan; 2017. Retrieved from: ibrary.ui.edu.ng/handle/123456789/4286

[13] Cerón A, Dillinger K, Eitniear M, Ernstrom S, Hedidar W, Hellinga C, et al. Global Kidney Exchange: Analysis and Background Papers from the Perspective of Medical Anthropology: Undergraduate Student Scholarship. 2. 2017. Available from: https://digitalcommons.du.edu/anthropology_student/2

[14] Kar D, Spanjers J. Transnational Crime and the Developing World. Washington: Global Financial Integrity; 2017. pp. 53-59

[15] Tao D. Worldwide market fuels illegal traffic in organs. 2009. New York Times, 29. Available from: https://www.manhassetschools.org/cms/lib/NY01913789/Centricity/Domain/272/Scarcity%20with%20Kidneys.pdf

[16] Sharif A, Singh MF, Trey T, Lavee J. Organ procurement from executed prisoners in China. American Journal of Transplantation. 2014;**14**(10):2246-2252

[17] Bruckmüller K. Trafficking of human beings for organ (cells and tissue) removal. In: Winterdyk J, Jones J, editors. The Palgrave International Handbook of Human Trafficking. Cham: Palgrave Macmillan; 2020:319-337. DOI: 10.1007/978-3-319-63058-8_20

[18] Bos M. Trafficking in Human Organs. EPRS: European Parliamentary Research Service. Directorate–generale for external policies, policy department; 2015. pp. 35-60. Retrieved from: https://policycommons.net/artifacts/1336189/trafficking-in-human-organs/1943170/ on 11 Sep 2022. CID: 20.500.12592/w19q85

[19] United Nations Office on Drugs and Crime. Assessment toolkit: Trafficking in Persons for the Purpose of Organ Removal. 2015. Available from: https://www.unodc.org/documents/human-trafficking/2015/UNODC_Assessment_Toolkit_TIP_for_the_Purpose_of_Organ_Removal.pdf

[20] Francis LP, Francis JG. Stateless crimes, legitimacy, and international criminal law: The case of organ trafficking. Criminal Law and Philosophy. 2010;**4**(3):283-295

[21] Adido TO. Enforcement of transplant tourism criminal law model. In: Transplant Tourism. The Netherlands: Leiden; 2018. pp. 222-262. DOI: 10.1163/9789004362772_008 Brill | Nijhoff

[22] Ambagtsheer F. Understanding the challenges to investigating and prosecuting organ trafficking: A comparative analysis of two cases. Trends in Organized Crime (June 2021). Sept 2022;**25**(3):1-28. DOI: 10.1007/s12117-021-09421-2

[23] Martin DE, Van Assche K, Domínguez-Gil B, López-Fraga M, García Gallont R, Muller E, et al. Strengthening global efforts to combat organ trafficking and transplant tourism: Implications of the 2018 Edaition of the declaration of Istanbul. Transplantation direct. 2019;**5**(3):e433. DOI: 10.1097/TXD.0000000000000872

[24] Kao A. The Physician's role in discussing organ donation at the end of life. AMA Journal of Ethics. 2000. DOI: 10.1001/virtualmentor.2000.2.12.elce1-0012. Available from: https://journalofethics.ama-assn.org/article/physicians-role-discussing-organ-donation-end-life/2000-12

[25] Thornton JD, Curtis JR, Allen MD. Completion of advanced care directives is associated with willingness to donate. Journal of the National Medical Association. 2006;**98**(6):897-904

[26] O'Carroll RE, Foster C, McGeechan G, Sandford K, Fergeson E. The "ick" factor, anticipated regret, and willingness to become an organ donor. Health Psychology. 2011;**30**(2):236-245

[27] US Department of Health and Human Services Health Resources and Services Administration Healthcare Systems Bureau. 2012 National Survey of Organ Donation Attitudes and Behaviors. Rockville, MD: US Department of Health and Human Services; 2013

[28] Caulfield T, Duijst W, Bos M, Chassis I, Codreanu I, Danovitch G, et al. Trafficking in human beings for the purpose of organ removal and the ethical and legal obligations of healthcare providers. Transplantation direct. 4 Jan 2016;**2**(2):e60. DOI: 10.1097/

TXD.000000'0000000566. PMID: 27500253; PMCID: PMC4946496

[29] Gawronska S, Claes L, Van Assche K. Double prosecution of illicit organ removal as organ trafficking and human trafficking, with the example of Belgium. European Journal on Criminal Policy and Research. 2020:1-2. DOI: 10.1007/s10610-020-09466-z

[30] de Jong J, Ambagtsheer F. Indicators to identify trafficking in human beings for the purpose of organ removal. Transplantation direct. 4 Jan 2016;**2**(2):e56. DOI: 10.1097/TXD.0000000000000568. PMID: 27500249; PMCID: PMC4946497

[31] Nullis-Kapp C. Organ trafficking and transplantation pose new challenges. Bulletin of the World Health Organization. 2004;**82**:715-715

[32] Zimik TN. Human trafficking in Northeast India. International Journal in Management & Social Science. 2015;**3**(6):263-269

[33] Okere ZC, Emedolu C. Issues on organ transplant: Ethical dimension. International Journal of Research Publication and Reviews. 2022;**3**:472-474

Chapter 6

Organ Donation in Islam

Sahar Khoshravesh

Abstract

Nowadays, the increasing scientific and practical advances in the field of organ donation have caused many discussions in the world. One of these topics is religious beliefs in divine religions, which has always been one of the most important challenges in the field of organ donation. Although there are differences in the views of different religions regarding organ donation, many of these views are close to each other. Often, different sects and religions have accepted organ transplantation with their own conditions. Based on Islamic jurisprudence and Shariah principles, organ donation is permissible under certain conditions; most religious scholars have also accepted this opinion. The Muslim holy book (Qur'an 5:32) has mentioned, "if anyone saved a life, it would be as if he saved the life of the whole people."

Keywords: organ donation, Islam, religion, religious, challenge

1. Introduction

From a long time ago, the connection of ethics and science in different fields of knowledge has always been an important and obvious principle for the material and spiritual advancement of mankind. In the realm of experimental sciences, especially medicine, ethics is considered an inseparable part. The principles of medical ethics have four principles, which Islam has also accepted. These four principles are as follows:

1. Autonomy: It means that the patient has the right to choose or refuse his treatment method.

2. Beneficence: It means that the person working in this field should act for the benefit of the patient and his benefit.

3. Non-maleficence: It means not harming a person.

4. Justice: It means issues related to the distribution of scarce health care resources and decisions about who receives what treatment, justice, fairness, and equality should be observed [1].

The emergence of Islam and its emphasis on scientific education and attention on medical science have had a great impact on the progress of science in Islamic countries. Almost all great Muslim doctors had full knowledge of theology and their works were both in the field of medicine and in the field of jurisprudence and ethics.

Islamic medical ethics are based on the principles of respecting human life and preserving its values. From the point of view of Islam, besides being a social necessity, and human and moral mission, medicine is also a Shariah responsibility, because it is obligatory for a man to reach the highest levels of human perfection. Considering that medical science deals with the treatment of disease and maintaining human health, the doctor should study the features and subtleties of the creation system in the body. Therefore, during the training period and even during the treatment, he is constantly dealing with the complexities of the existential system. For these reasons, the medical profession connects man with God more than other professions.

In the medical profession, it is necessary to keep in mind the following four general principles that Islam has in mind about a man and his life in all medical matters, so that we can make the right decision more easily when making a decision for each person.

a. Belief in the purposeful life of all human beings.

b. Belief in the value of every person's life.

c. Belief in the existence of individual differences.

d. Belief in the ability and readiness of each person to do things according to their abilities.

In addition to paying attention to medical issues, medical scientists have also given ethical recommendations. The teachings of Islam have advised Muslim scientists to have commitment and responsibility in medicine, to acquire expertise, be careful in their work, avoid any negligence in the matter of medicine, and pay attention to the mental and physical health of patients as the most important points of medical ethics in prophetic medicine. All the scientists of the world believe in the Hippocratic Oath in medicine. With a little possession, this oath is known as the "Oath of a Muslim Doctor" in the view of Islamic doctors. This oath, which is a mixture of the moral teachings of Hippocrates and Islamic culture, contains the following points:

- Paying full attention to performing sensitive medical duties;
- Effort in treating and guiding patients;
- Considering the sanctity and spirituality of medicine in strengthening the morale and maintaining the health of patients;
- Avoiding contaminating the sanctity of medicine with unstable material symptoms and sensual moods and satanic temptations;
- Respect for divine decrees and limits;
- Serious avoidance of betrayal and violation of patients' rights; keeping patients' secrets except in cases of necessity;
- Knowing that God is present and watching in all situations.

2. Islam view about scientific progress in the organ donation field

In Islam, science and practice are tied together with religious and moral values. Islam has welcomed science and scientific research, and has always encouraged Muslims to strive for scientific progress and excellence.

Organ transplantation is one of the new issues of medical science and one of its important achievements. The brain death phenomenon and the possibility of using it in organ transplantation, although it has brought new hopes in saving the lives of a number of patients, it has also brought many moral, cultural, and legal issues. In Islamic sources, human life is sacred, and preserving his life is a divine duty [2, 3]. Islam's attention on new scientific research and findings in meeting the religious and worldly needs of man gives legitimacy to medical advances in saving human lives.

Efforts to remove obstacles and problems in organ transplantation, in addition to reducing the costs of maintaining brain-dead patients and giving hope to patients in need of organ transplantation, prevent profit-seeking, and unethical and illegal actions in this field. Since the culture that governs the Islamic society is an authentic Islamic culture, medical innovations and procedures, including organ transplantation, must be in accordance with Islamic standards and pay special attention to moral issues and problems in the Islamic society, otherwise failure in experience. Because even if this issue is legal, people will withdraw as the main provider and will not accept organ transplants due to moral problems.

3. Religious beliefs related to organ donation in Islam

Today, the increasing scientific and practical advances in the field of organ donation have caused many discussions in the world. One of these topics is religious beliefs in divine religions, which has always been one of the most important challenges in the field of organ donation. Although there are differences in the views of different religions regarding organ donation, many of these views are close to each other. Often, different sects and religions have accepted organ transplantation with their own conditions [4].

Given that the issue of organ donation and organ transplantation close communication with humans and their life and also religions, moral philosophies and different social traditions have different views about man, body, and soul. So, the issue of organ transplantation has been the source of many ethical, philosophical, and legal debates in the world. The views of religions on this issue are often related to the place of man in their value system. Because organ transplantation is closely related to the human body and decisions related to it. For example, in Islam, any action that is considered to treat and save human life is accepted. As in the Muslim holy book (Qur'an 5:32) is clearly mentioned, "if anyone saved a life, it would be as if he saved the life of the whole people" [4].

Religion and religious beliefs are one of the important and effective aspects of organ donation, because religion and religious beliefs are very influential in the cultural structure of societies, people's thinking, and performance in various fields [4]. In the term, religion is a worldview and a set of beliefs that try to provide an explanation for a series of questions that are created for humans throughout their life [5].

Paying attention to religious beliefs is one of the main matters that make people consider organ donation as a pious and good act that brings them closer to God.

Because every brain death victim can save several patients who need organs from inevitable death. It must be acknowledged that accepting organ donation is a moral, godly, and altruistic act, and all societies should try to spread this beautiful act [6].

Evidence shows that the relationship between Islamic teachings and organ donation is very complex. Religious beliefs, especially Islamic beliefs, may be considered as both barriers and facilitators of organ donation. On the one hand, Islam attaches great importance to preserving human life, so that by supporting organ donation, it has been able to provide an opportunity to create a positive public atmosphere to promote the culture of organ donation in Islamic countries (Qur'an 5:32). On the other hand, some Muslims based on views, such as that God is the protector of human life and the process of life preservation and treatment is in his hands, do not believe in organ donation for the treatment of diseases that require organ donation or do not accept organ donation because they believe that removing body parts is a kind of respect for the dead body.

Positive religious beliefs regarding organ donation can have a profound effect on improving public attitudes and lead to an increase in organ donation in society, although most people do not have sufficient knowledge regarding religious issues in the field of organ donation. It seems that in intervention studies related to increasing organ donation, special attention should be paid to increasing people's awareness of correct religious beliefs and correcting incorrect religious beliefs. In a recent intervention study in Iran, it was tried not only to increase people's awareness about correct religious beliefs, but also to correct wrong religious beliefs. For example, some people think that it was God's will that a person needs a transplant, so there is no need for doctors to do anything to save him, or they think that God's will is that the body is buried healthy after death. Therefore, it is important to correct such false religious beliefs [7].

The presence of religious beliefs, such as the inevitability of death, being alive after death, and the continued existence after death in Muslims, encourages them to donate organs. For example, based on the religious teachings of Islam, Muslims do not emphasize on maintaining the integrity of the body, because Muslims believe that after death, the human body will be rebuilt in the resurrection.

In Islam, man is the best of creation and the God's Caliph on earth (Qur'an 1:30). Man has been given reason and free will, and man is not only responsible for his health, but he must also strive to preserve his life. God has respected human life in the Qur'an (5:32), so that this verse clearly legitimizes medical advances in saving human lives and prohibits suicide and euthanasia. Muslims due to Islamic teachings, emphasizing the importance of saving a human life, are encouraged to save a human life. Islamic teachings have a key role in persuading Muslims to save human life and this view can influence the positive public attitudes toward organ donation [8].

4. The jurisprudential ruling of donating organs in the Islamic perspective

The jurisprudential ruling of transplanting/donating organs is one of the major concerns of Islamic societies, and contemporary jurists have presented different interpretations according to the verses, hadiths, and examination of jurisprudential texts and rules. Some believe that it is not permissible to transplant organs, and others consider it permissible with some restrictions and conditions.

Therefore, it is natural to answer the following questions:

- What is Islam's opinion on organ donation?

- Where does this opinion come from?
- Does Islam have obstacles or conditions for this matter and if it has obstacles or conditions, in which case?

First of all, the general framework of the cognition of humans from the Islamic viewpoint on organ donation should be defined, because when God sent his prophets to convey the divine message to the people, they all had a basic concern. Their only concern has been to solve the spiritual, physical, moral, psychological, and livelihood problems of man and lead him to progress and excellence.

Within the scope of the human-to-human relationship, the special concern of Islam has been to bring man out of the cocoon of his individuality toward philanthropy, forgiveness, and self-sacrifice in order to obtain the mercy and grace of God. Regarding the Islamic society, the Holy Prophet of Islam says: "The example of the believers in terms of compassion and kindness among themselves is like the members of a body, if one part of it hurts, the rest of the members sympathize with him by waking up at night."

In the religion of Islam, the highest form of forgiveness is to prefer others over oneself, so that the benefit of others is preferred over one's benefit and their comfort is preferred over one's comfort. So, self-sacrifice is the best form of worship and the highest degree of faith.

Therefore, due to the fact that forgiveness and self-sacrifice are at the heart of Islam religion, we can understand that organ donation in Islam has a special sanctity and encourages Muslims to donate organs. According to Islamic jurisprudence and Shariah principles, organ donation is permissible under certain conditions. Most religious scholars and jurisprudential communities have also accepted this opinion. The most obvious of these conditions are stated below:

-In organ donation from a living person to a living person, the donor must be aware of what he is doing and do it voluntarily. Organ donation should not cause the death of the donor or failure of his vital and necessary organs, such as eyes, heart, or other vital organs. Because the rule of jurisprudence says: a loss cannot be removed by a similar loss [9].

- Religious affiliations of the donor, his kinship ties, and gender should not be considered.
- If organ donation occurs after the death of the donor, organ donation should be done with the consent of the patient's family.
- Respecting a dead person is like a living person. Therefore, it is necessary to take all necessary precautions to preserve the respect of the dead body after taking the required organ and then burying the dead body according to Sharia standards [10].

5. Some reasons for agreeing to organ donation

In the following, some of the most important reasons for those who agree with removing organs from people with brain death in Islamic society are stated:

5.1 The vital role of transplant in preserving human life

From the verses of the Holy Qur'an and many hadiths, as well as the words of religious scholars, this point is well used that saving a life is especially important.

However, many haram actions are considered permissible in case of conflict with the preservation of one's own or another's life. Therefore, in the confrontation between saving the life of a Muslim and the prohibition of dissection, the saving of a Muslim's life can be prioritized over the prohibition of dissection. In the case of organ transplantation, saving the life of a Muslim takes precedence over the dissection of another Muslim's body, and its haram status is removed.

5.2 Relieving the hardships of patients who need organ transplants

The lack of transplanted organs and ethically acceptable ways to provide the needed organs to patients who need organ transplants are among the most important issues in this field. As we know, many patients who need a transplant die while waiting for a transplant, and they had a hard life before they died. Now, if it is possible to transplant these patients, they can return to normal life and be rescued from suffering and hardship [11].

6. Some reasons for disagreeing to organ donation

Although the religion of Islam agrees with the issue of organ donation, still some people in Islamic societies are against organ donation. Below are some of them.

6.1 Insulting the dead

The main reason for the opponents of organ harvesting from people with brain death and transplanting it to needy patients is that dismembering the dead body and cutting his organs is an insult to the dignity of the dead. In fact, the opponents believe that the practice of organ transplantation actually calls into question the respect we give to the dead bodies [11].

Burial ceremonies are a common custom in all human societies, and forbidding people from such ceremonies is considered as a great insult to human identity. Particularly if the deceased is a Muslim, which according to some hadiths, the obligation to respect a Muslim is not limited to his lifetime, and respect for him is also necessary while he is dying and he should not be insulted. In response to this argument, it should be said that these hadiths are used as long as the necessity does not require it, and there is nothing more important than respecting Muslims. If the harvesting of the body parts of Muslim preserves the respect of the Muslim, and the saving of the life of the Muslim or Muslims depends on the removing of the organ from the dead Muslim and transplanting it to the patients, then it is permissible.

6.2 Not accepting brain death as absolute death

A brain death person has life and is not yet completely dead, so organ transplantation is unallowable.

In response to this issue, it should be said that nowadays brain death is considered absolute death in medicine. Accepting this, especially for those who have an emotional connection with a person who has suffered brain death, while he has a pulse, is breathing, his complexion is normal, and he appears to have just fallen into a deep sleep, it is very difficult. It is obvious that if brain death is not considered a definite death, organ transplantation from brain-dead people, which is a great source of organ supply, will face a serious problem. By dividing the stages of life into the full life of the corpse, continuous vegetative life, life of organs and cell life, and dissection, we all come to the conclusion that human death occurs in three stages:

1. Stopping the activity of the heart and lungs.

2. Death of brain cells after a few minutes of deprivation of receiving oxygen-carrying blood.

3. The death of the cells of the body, which is different compared with the organs.

This arrangement exists in the state of natural death, but in the state of brain death, death from the second stage. That is, the death of brain cells starts and consequently leads to the cessation of the activity of the heart and lungs and finally the death of the cells [12].

6.3 Violation of the creation system rules

Extending human life through organ transplantation is a problem that may be considered in conflict with Godly views. With this approach, we finally understand that new technologies have forced us to sometimes reflect on this question. Can the laws of Islamic society contradict what we know as the laws of nature, including respect to customs, such as family ties and religious-cultural values?

Some Buddhist groups also believe that prolonging human life by accepting another person's organ or body through organ transplantation is unnatural and immoral. Also, waiting for others to die in order to continue living is immoral in their view.

This argument is also not acceptable due to the fact that maintaining health, preventing disease, and treating disease are logical axioms, and Sharia has approved it, even considered it obligatory. Therefore, the use of treatment methods with respect to divine limits is desirable and necessary [11].

6.4 Misuse of the organs

Another reason for the opponents of organ donation is the possibility of possible misuse, such as the buying and selling of organs of brain-dead patients by some doctors, profiteers, and even the rich people. The opponents believe that the following may occur:

1. Doctors do not use sufficient accuracy in prioritizing between the organ recipient and the donor, they pay less attention to the medical issues and consequences of transplantation, and in fact, the first word in the prioritization is the trading of organs, the criterion of which will be the payment of more money.

2. By paying the fee on behalf of those who have more income, the price of the organs of brain death patients increases day by day, and as a result, it causes deprivation of poor families from transplanted organs.

3. Allowing the buying and selling of organs in a region can attract rich people to trade in transplanted organs and may have uncontrollable consequences.

In response, it should be said that the existing problems cannot be a valid reason for prohibiting the use of the organs of brain death patients. Rather, it requires control and consideration of logical solutions, because sometimes the treatment of some chronic diseases is only possible through organ transplantation [11].

6.5 Having negative social consequences

Accepting permission to remove organs for transplantation and recommending it causes negative social consequences, many of which will not be controllable. For example, it is possible that the removal of organs is not limited to the ones that exist now, and other organs that have other interests are removed and there is nothing left of the human being to be buried.

In response to this issue, it should be said that if we can prevent this problem by establishing the necessary regulations and precautions, this certainly cannot be a reason for prohibiting organ donation, as currently in various countries only organ donation is permitted. It is not enough, but special regulations have been considered for the organization of organ donation, removal, and transplantation [11].

Below are the details of organ donation law in Iran as one of the Islamic countries.

In Iran, the organ donation program was established after Imam Khomeini's jurisprudence supported the use of organs from deceased donors in 2000.

In this year, the organ transplant law was approved by Islamic Consultative Assembly [13]. The text of this law is as follows:

Hospitals equipped for transplanting organs, after obtaining written permission from the Ministry of Health, Treatment and Medical Education, can use the healthy organs of deceased patients or patients whose brain death is certain according to the opinion of experts, on the condition of the patient's will or the consent of the deceased's guardian for transplantation for patients whose survival depends on transplanting the above-mentioned organs or organs.

Note 1: Diagnosis of brain death is done by experts in equipped hospitals of state universities. These experts are appointed by the decree of the Minister of Health, Treatment and Medical Education for four years.

Note 2: The members of brain death detection teams should not be members of transplant teams.

Note 3: The doctors who are members of the team will not be included in the payment of ransom due to the injuries inflicted on the deceased.

It should be noted that Sunni scholars also have an acceptable consensus in the field of organ donation. For example, in 1982, the Sunni Scholars Association issued a fatwa on the permissibility of organ transplantation. Other fatwas have been issued in this regard.

In a conference held in 1989, some Islamic scholars, while pointing to the respect for the human body and stressing on not harming the human body (dead or alive), have pointed out that it is permissible to use the human body in a way that pleases God.

7. Diversity of views in different religions about organ donation

As we said before, the role of religious beliefs in organ donation is undeniable. Although there are differences in specific views, it is obvious that most religions in the world permit and support transplantation and donation. In the following, some of these views are expressed.

- **AME & AME Zion**
  Organ donation is a charity act and a way of helping others.
- **Amish**
  They agree with transplantation if there is definite evidence that the recipient's health will improve.
- **Assembly of God**
  The church has no official policy about donation. The decision to donate is up to the individual.
- **Baptist**
  Donation is supported as an act of charity and the church leaves the decision to donate up to the individual.
- **Brethren**
  In the Brethren's Annual Conference in 1993 about the support of organ donation has been mentioned that "We have the opportunity to help others out of love for Christ, through the donation of organs and tissues."
- **Buddhism**
  Buddhists believe that organ donation is an individual conscience act. They highlight the importance of letting family members inform one's desires about organ donation.
- **Catholicism**
  Organ donation is acceptable to the Vatican and this is supported as an act of charity and love.
- **Christian church**
  The Christian Church persuades organ donation. Their belief is that humans were created for God's glory and for sharing God's love.
- **Episcopal**
  A resolution has passed by the Episcopal Church about the benefits of organ, tissue, and blood donation in 1982. All Christians are encouraged to become organ and blood donors.
- **Greek Orthodox**
  The Greek Orthodox Church has no opposition to organ donation as long as the organ donation is used to better the life of human.
- **Gypsies**
  The Gypsies believe that for one year after death, the soul retraces its steps. So, the body must remain complete because the soul sustains its physical shape.
- **Hinduism**
  Organ donation is an individual decision. It is not in contrast to the Hindu religion.

- **Independent conservative evangelical**
  In general, Evangelicals have no objection to organ donation, and this is an individual decision.

- **Islam**
  Although the generality of transplanting organs from the organs of brain death patients is accepted in both Shia and Sunni religions in Islam, still some authorities of these two religions do not agree with organ donation, and their most important problem is the lack of belief in brain death as definitive death.

- **Jehovah's witnesses**
  Organ donation is an individual conscience issue with the provision that all organs of the body be completely drained of blood.

- **Judaism**
  Jews emphasize that if it is possible to donate an organ to save a life, it is mandatory to do.

- **Lutheran**
  A resolution has passed by the Lutheran Church in America about the role of organ donation in the well-being of humanity in 1984. They invite "members to pay attention to organ donation and to make any necessary family and legal preparation, like the sign donor card."

- **Mennonite**
  Mammonites have no formal position on organ donation, but are not opposed to it. They emphasize the decision to donate is related to the individual and/or their family.

- **Pentecostal**
  They believe that the decision to donate should be left up to the individual.

- **Presbyterian**
  Presbyterians support organ donation. They respect an individual's right to make decisions about their own body.

- **Protestantism**
  The Protestantism supports and encourages organ donation.

- **Seventh-Day Adventist**
  Organ donation/transplantation is strongly supported by Seventh-Day Adventists.

- **Society of friends**
  The Society of Friends does not have an official position on donation. Donation is an individual decision.

- **Unitarian Universalist**
  Organ donation is generally supported by Unitarian Universalists. They believe that an organ donation is an act of love and selfless giving.

- **United Church of Christ**
  The United Church of Christ encourages donation.

- **United Methodist**
  The United Methodist Church passed a policy statement about organ donation. The United Methodist Church emphasizes the benefits of organ donation and encourages all Christians to become organ donors [14].

Key points

- The role of religious beliefs in organ donation is undeniable. Although there are variations in specific views, it is obvious that most religions in the world permit and support transplantation and donation.

- Religion and religious beliefs are one of the important and effective aspects of organ donation. Because there are very influential in the cultural structure of societies, people's thinking, and performance in various fields.

- Positive religious beliefs regarding organ donation can have a profound effect on improving public attitudes and lead to an increase in organ donation in society.

- In Islam, any action that is considered to treat and save human life is accepted. Based on the Muslim holy book (Qur'an 5:32), "if anyone saved a life, it would be as if he saved the life of the whole people."

- According to Islamic jurisprudence and Shariah principles, organ donation is permissible under certain conditions. Most religious scholars have also accepted this opinion.

- Some reasons for disagreeing with organ donation are insulting the dead, not accepting brain death as absolute death, violation of the creation system rules, misuse of the organs, and having negative social consequences.

Author details

Sahar Khoshravesh
Department of Public Health, Hamadan University of Medical Sciences, Hamadan, Iran

*Address all correspondence to: edu.umsha.ac.ir

References

[1] Gillon R. Medical ethics: Four principles plus attention to scope. BMJ (Clinical research ed). 1994;**309**(6948):184-188

[2] Daar AS. Prospects of organ sharing and strategies for increasing transplants in Asia. Transplantation Proceedings. 1998;**30**(7):3649

[3] Sque M, Payne S, Vlachonikolis I. Cadaveric donotransplantation: Nurses' attitudes, knowledge and behaviour. Social Science & Medicine. 1982;**52**(4): 541-552

[4] Kajian O, Islami H, Ashkazari MRD. Identifying Barriers and Motivational Factors of Religious Culture of Organ Donation in TV Programs. 2021

[5] Manzari ZS, Mohammadi E, Heidari A. Factors influencing organ donation decisions by brain death patients' families: A qualitative study. Payesh. 2012;**11**(6):913-925

[6] Khani L, Hashemianfar A, Ghaffari M, Smaili R, Ansari E. Designing an organ donation model based on variables of social ethics, altruism, and religiousness. Religion and Health. 2016;**4**(1):1-11

[7] Khoshravesh S, Karimi-Shahanjarini A, Poorolajal J, Barati M, Bashirian S, Hamidi M, et al. Evaluation of a workplace organ donation intervention: A randomized controlled trial. Journal of Community and Applied Social Psychology. 2021

[8] Hejazi SS, Nikbakht S, Jouybari L, Abadi MH, Davoodi D, Azizi TH, et al. Knowledge and attitudes toward brain death and organ donation in Bojnurd. Electronic Physician. 2017;**9**(7):4746-4752

[9] Nazafarin G, Fariba A, Mandana S, Fatemeh Faramarzi R, Bagher L. Islamic jurisprudential and ethical considerations of practicing medical procedures on nearly dead patients: Part II (Shiite jurisprudents' viewpoints). Journal of Medical Ethics and History of Medicine. 2015;**11**:6

[10] Donating Organs from a Jurisprudential Point of View/5 Possible Obstacles in Donating Organs to Others. Available from: http://vasael.ir/fa/news/14951/. 2019

[11] MotahariPour M. Ethical consideration in organ transplantation. Research Quarterly in Islamic Ethics. 2013;**6**(19):119-136

[12] Seraji M. The nature of brain death from the viewpoint of Quran and Hadith. Arak Medical University Journal. 2011;**13**(5):65-77

[13] Afzal Aghaee M, Dehghani M, Sadeghi M, Khaleghi E. Awareness of religious leaders' fatwa and willingness to donate organ. International Journal of Organ Transplantation Medicine. 2015;**6**(4):158-164

[14] https://www.kidney.org/atoz/content/religion-organ-donation

Section 3

Advances in Organ Donation

Chapter 7

Recent Advances and Outcomes in Heart and Lung Transplantation

Akshay Kumar, Sania Thite, Varad Wazarkar, Kamal Ayyat, Jesus Gomez Abraham and Suresh Keshavamurthy

Abstract

Heart and lung transplantations are established treatments for patients with end-stage heart and lung failure, respectively. As mechanical circulatory devices, extracorporeal membrane oxygenation, organ perfusion, and transport systems advance, so do patient comorbidities and profiles of patients undergoing transplantation are becoming more complex. With the ever-increasing shortage of donor organs, marginal and high-risk donor utilization continues to rise. In this chapter, we attempt to elucidate the recent advances and outcomes in heart and lung transplantation. We also highlight how an ongoing COVID-19 pandemic affects the logistics of transplant programs.

Keywords: donation after circulatory death, ischemia–reperfusion injury, organ care systems, *ex vivo* lung perfusion, COVID-19

1. Introduction

Each year, more than 4500 lung transplants are performed worldwide, over 2500 of which occur in North America itself [1]. The year 2020 faced unique challenges due to the onslaught of the COVID-19 pandemic. Social distancing, physical isolation, and travel restrictions made people increasingly hesitant to seek healthcare as hospitals were overburdened with COVID-19 patients. As the accessibility to healthcare declined, fewer candidates were added to the waitlist, and even fewer underwent a transplant. Additions to the waitlist saw a 17% decline from 2019 [2]. Procurement of organs from eligible donors was further complicated by travel bans. The dip in donor availability and infrequent healthcare access by transplant candidates ultimately led to a rise in waitlist mortality from 14.7 deaths per 100 waitlist years in 2019 to 16.1 in 2020 [2]. For those who were scheduled to receive a transplant, the health risks posed by the virus on the already frail lung transplant recipients were a major concern. In time, it was noticed that some COVID-19-infected patients could develop end-stage lung disease, which itself could require lung transplantation. Consequently, in the early half of 2021, 165 patients underwent transplantation for COVID-19 infection [2]. Another complexity was COVID-19 infection among donors. While it was initially viewed apprehensively, studies were conducted to assess the impact of transplanting organs from COVID-19-infected donors to healthy recipients. Although

IntechOpen

statistics did not disclose any impact on the early survival rates, more long-term studies are necessary [3]. Recently, Eichenberger et al. reported the safe and effective use of hearts from COVID-19-positive donors. 14 thoracic transplants in 13 recipients were performed using organs from COVID-19-positive donors. None of the recipients or healthcare members acquired COVID-19. No recipients suffered unexpected acute rejection. Patient survival was 92% to date, with graft survival 93% [4].

2. Lung-recipient characteristics

Survival among lung transplant recipients has remained stable in 2020 despite the effects of the COVID-19 pandemic as compared with the previous year. The 1-year survival was close to 90% . 61.2% of recipients who underwent a transplant in 2015 survived for 5 years, and 33.1% of recipients from 2010 survived for 10 years. When comparing within age groups, the 5-year survival was lowest for recipients aged 65 and older [2].

Due to a more inclusive candidate profile, we see a corresponding shift in the recipient characteristics. The past decade boasts of the inclusion of a larger age and BMI group as compared to the 1990s with the median age increasing to 57 from 50, and the median BMI rising from 25.0 kg/m2 to 26.5 kg/m2 [5]. As more patients have comorbidities, the patient profile is increasingly complex. The proportion of lung transplant recipients having diabetes mellitus has seen a sharp rise. Between 2010 and 2018, 20.1% of recipients had diabetes. This figure was only 6.1% as recorded in Oct 1999–Dec 2000. Patients with malignancies have also become more frequent. 7.9% of lung transplant recipients had a history of malignancy in 2010–2018 as compared to only 2.7% between 1994 and 2000 [5]. A similar trend is noted in recipients of heart transplants. Patients have increased BMI, and a greater percentage suffer from comorbidities, such as diabetes and malignancies [5].

Traditionally, lung transplants in adults have been performed mainly for chronic obstructive pulmonary disease (COPD), idiopathic interstitial pneumonia (IIP),

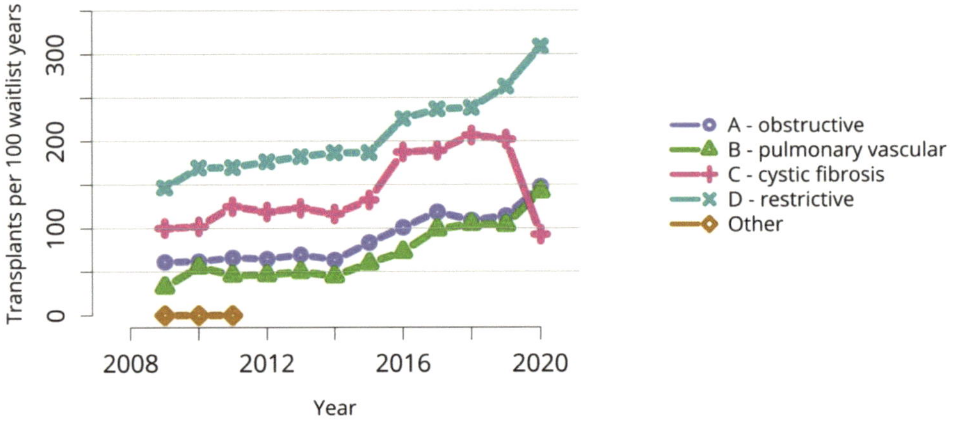

Figure 1.
Deceased donor lung transplant rates among adult waitlist candidates by diagnosis group. Transplant rates are computed as the number of deceased donor transplants per 100 patient-years of wait time in a given year. Individual listings are counted separately. The other/unknown group includes a small number of heart-lung candidates prior to 2015 who did not have an a/B/C/D diagnosis group specified. (from OPTN/SRTR 2020 annual data report. HHS/HRSA).

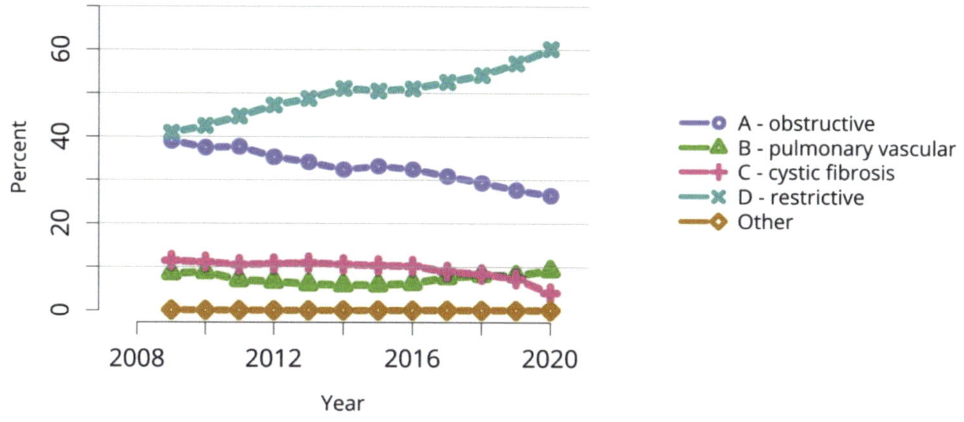

Figure 2.
Distribution of adults waiting for lung transplant by diagnosis group. Candidates waiting for a transplant at any time in the given year. Candidates listed at more than one center are counted once per listing. Active and inactive patients are included. The other/unknown group includes a small number of heart-lung candidates prior to 2015 who did not have an a/B/C/D diagnosis group specified. (from OPTN/SRTR 2020 annual data report. HHS/HRSA.)

and cystic fibrosis (CF). These formed 30.1%, 26.1%, and 15.2% of all transplants respectively from Jan 1995 to June 2018 [6]. The year 2020 saw a sharp decline in the transplants done for cystic fibrosis due to patient stabilization following cystic fibrosis transmembrane conductance regulator (CFTR) modulator therapy (**Figure 1**). Nevertheless, cystic fibrosis remains the number 1 indication for a lung transplant in the pediatric age group [2]. The OPTN/SRTR 2020 annual data report reflects a study rise in lung transplants performed for patients suffering from restrictive lung diseases, from 263.0 transplants per 100 waitlist years in 2019 to 308.7 in 2020. On the contrary, among adults waiting for a lung transplant, a decline is seen in patients needing transplants for obstructive lung disease (**Figure 2**).

3. Lung-donation after circulatory death

With the continued shortage of donor's lungs, donation after circulatory death (DCD) has emerged as an option in addition to conventional brain dead (BD) donation to increase the donor pool. Patients with extensive and devastating brain injury where the damage is recognized to be irreversible but who are not brain dead qualify as a potential donor, if by advance directives or family consent it is decided to withdraw life support (WLST). After withdrawal of support, death is usually declared after a 5–15-min window of no cardiac activity also called a stand-off period. In the most recent era, DCD organ use comprise 4.2% of all lung transplants. Recipient outcomes from DCD donors are equivalent to BD donors. The Maastricht classification defines DCD categories (classes I-V) according to the circumstances of the donor's death. Controlled DCD (class III) includes patients who cannot be resuscitated and undergo WLST following cardiac arrest, determination, and organ donation [7]. Cypel et al. from Toronto described their simple method of *in situ* donor lung preservation for uDCD (uncontrolled DCD) where, in contrast to most of the European experience, no reinstitution of circulation (via normothermic regional perfusion or continuous chest compressions) is performed after cardiac arrest and death declaration, and only simple measures of lung protection are initiated. Of 30 cases consented for uDCD, donor's lungs were retrieved from 16 donors, the remaining 14 lungs ultimately underwent EVLP to evaluate suitability for transplant; finally, lungs from five donors were used—four bilateral lungs and one left single-lung transplant (16.7% utilization rate from consented donors) [8].

4. Expanding the donor pool with increased-risk donors

As the criteria for the candidacy for lung transplantation keeps evolving [9], the number of people awaiting a transplant is also increasing. Based on the organ procurement & transplantation network (OPTN) Metrics, by the 52nd week of 2021, the cumulative waitlist total for lung transplantation was 3091, but only 2631 donors could be recovered. This ultimately resulted in a total of 2524 lung transplants in 2021. Due to the ever-increasing shortage of donors, expanding the donor pool has become necessary. In addition to traditional donors, strategies are now in place to procure organs from increased risk donors (IRD), which help in closing the gap substantially. In 2013, the United States Public Health Service categorized organ donors with risk factors for human immunodeficiency virus (HIV), hepatitis B virus (HBV), or hepatitis C virus (HCV) as IRDs [10].

4.1 ODD and HCV-positive donors

The ongoing opioid crisis in the United States has caused an increase in the number of overdose-related deaths, consequently increasing the number of overdose-death donors (ODD). The proportion of ODDs increased from 1.1% in 2000 to 13.4% in 2017, while trauma-death donors (TDD) and medical-death donors (MDD) saw only a marginal increase of 1.6% per year and 2.3% per year, respectively [11].

There were two major concerns with accepting organs from ODDs—the unknown outcomes, and the possibility of them being increased risk donors (IRD). Studies have measured the 1-year and 5-year survival rates after transplant for ODDs and have found that they are non-inferior as against TDDs and MDDs, which has helped attenuate the fear regarding uncertain outcomes [11]. The only remaining concern is the risk of transmission of blood-borne viruses, as a 30% prevalence of HCV among ODDs is a fairly apprehensive number [11]. The advent of direct-acting antivirals (DAA), and the availability of additional diagnostic means like nucleic acid testing (NAT), virus-specific antigens, and antibodies have offered some hope for better detection and reduction of transmission of these infections to the recipient [12].

With pretransplant mortality of 16.1 deaths per 100 waitlist years [2], there is an ever-growing need to find acceptable donor lungs. Studies have tried to assess the impact of transplanting lungs from HCV-positive donors on the waitlist numbers and post-transplant survival. Since DAAs have almost 97% HCV cure rates, several researchers have also tested the outcomes of transplanting lungs from HCV+ donors to HCV- recipients, after covering the recipient with a short course of DAAs. Patient and graft survival at 6 and 12 months have been like transplanting lungs from HCV- donors, but the odds of having acute rejection were higher in the HCV+ donor subgroup [13]. Viral load in recipients after transplantation and establishment of active HCV infection has also been researched. While some studies show undetectable HCV viral load post solid organ transplant, others have documented the establishment of infection [14, 15]. Some studies express concern over the possibility of false negative NAT and serologic testing in IRD, as seen during a window period because cases have been recorded demonstrating transmission of HCV infection during transplantation [16]. Nevertheless, with the increasing utilization of IRD lungs to the extent of 95%, HCV-positive donors potentially help shorten the donor-waitlist gap considerably [2]. While this approach shows promising results, long-term studies are needed to assess the impact on the quality of life of the recipients. Emerging modalities, such as *ex vivo* lung perfusion, have also led to the discovery of novel means to inactivate infections in allografts before transplantation.

5. HIV organ policy equity act

The signing of the HIV organ policy equity (HOPE) act into law in 2013 was a revolutionary move in expanding the organ donor pool as it enabled HIV-positive patients well-controlled on highly active antiretroviral therapy (HAART) to be registered as organ donors. People living with HIV (PLWH) are always at a higher risk of end-stage organ disease, more so because HAART has significantly reduced the rates of deadly opportunistic infections. Until recently, having an HIV infection was considered a contraindication for receiving a lung transplant [17]. Researchers have since found out that lung transplant survival rates and postoperative outcomes were similar in HIV-positive recipients as compared to their uninfected counterparts [18, 19]. Solid organ transplantation has therefore become the standard of care for organ failure in PLWH [20]. After clearing the way for HIV-positive transplant recipients, the HOPE act went one step ahead by allowing HIV-positive people to donate their organs to fellow individuals sharing their HIV-positive status.

Once the HOPE act was implemented in 2015, HIV-positive recipients began receiving organs from HIV-positive donors (HIV D+/R+). As of July 2021, there have been 144 true/false HIV-positive donors, which led to 300 kidney and 87 liver transplants [20]. This decision did not pass without its fair share of concerns. Healthcare professionals were worried about several plausible issues upon such transplants, particularly superinfection if the donor's HIV strain did not match the recipients, rate of rejection, and HIV-related organ disease in the allograft [21–23]. As compared to transplanting organs from HIV-negative donor to HIV-positive recipient (HIV D−/R+), the outcomes were similar, with the only real challenge being increased rates of rejection [24].

Heart and lung transplants from HIV-positive donors have been approved and are highly anticipated [20]. Federal HOPE Act guidelines require participating hospitals to carry out five transplants in HIV-positive recipients before they can accept organs from HIV-positive donors. Successful implementation of the HOPE act requires the address of community-level barriers like the lack of awareness, fear of infection in personnel procuring organs from HIV-positive patients, and the fear of revelation of donor/recipient HIV status during transplantation [25]. Challenges faced while coadministering HAART and immunosuppressive therapy also need to be considered. Such studies would lay the foundation for the successful initiation of thoracic organ transplants in HIV-infected individuals from HIV-positive donors. Koval et al. reported outcomes from 29 HIV-infected thoracic transplant recipients (21 heart, 7 lungs, and 1 heart and/or lung) across 14 transplant centers from 2000 through 2016. Compared to an ISHLT registry cohort, similar 1-, 3- and 5-year patient and allograft survival was seen. However, at 1 year, significant rejection rates were high (62%) for heart transplant recipients (HTRs). Pulmonary bacterial infections were high (86%) for lung transplant recipients (LTRs) [19].

6. *Ex vivo* lung perfusion (EVLP)

Ex vivo lung perfusion is a technique that allows harvested donor lungs to be explanted into a system that mimics the hemodynamic status of the human body. The general design of the system involves ventilation of the allograft via endotracheal tubes and circulation of a fraction of cardiac output by means of pumps [26]. In cellular EVLP protocols like the lund protocol and organ care system, packed red blood cells mixed with a composite perfusate are allowed to flow through the lungs, while acellular EVLP protocols like toronto protocol do not use blood cells in the perfusate [27]. It enables the assessment of hemodynamic, ventilatory, and gas exchange parameters of the allograft. Biochemical values, imaging studies, bronchoscopic analysis, physical inspection, and palpation can also be performed on these organs [26]. These factors allow EVLP to be used as a tool for analyzing the allograft before transplantation, which is especially useful in the case of marginal lungs facing the threat of being rejected. EVLP thus aims to maximize the utilization of procured donor lungs [26]. In cellular EVLP, Kamal et al. described direCt lung ultrasound evaluation (CLUE) technique as a method for monitoring extravascular lung water in donor lungs during *ex vivo* lung perfusion (EVLP). Significant differences were found between suitable and non-suitable lungs in CLUE scores (1.03 vs. 1.85, $p < 0.001$), unlike the partial pressure of oxygen/fraction of inspired oxygen ratio. Standard donors had significantly better scores than marginal lungs and proning improved this score, especially in upper lobes [28].

EVLP was mainly developed to tackle the problem of ischemic-reperfusion injury, which increases the risk of development of primary graft dysfunction (PGD) [29]. The current practice involves cold preservation of allografts that facilitates a reduction in the organ's metabolic demand. However, concerns regarding cold ischemic injury have surfaced. EVLP revolves around the principle of retaining the organ in its physiological milieu, at the human body temperature, for as long as possible [26]. Posttransplant outcomes after using EVLP have been consistently similar to traditional techniques in terms of patient and graft survival [30].

While the main role of EVLP remains the analysis of the graft, it is being creatively used to recondition the graft and even make initially rejected organs useful. In edematous lungs, EVLP allows the fluid from extravascular compartments to be drawn out, which can make the graft usable [31]. Antibiotics can be administered in the EVLP system, which ensures targeted therapy, preventing systemic adverse effects [32]. To shift the cytokine profile from pro-inflammatory to anti-inflammatory, Interleukin (IL)-10 gene therapy and stem cell therapies have been tried in porcine models by administering them to the graft using the EVLP systems [26].

Keeping in view the potential of eliminating infections from donor organs, trials began on organs harvested from HCV+ donors. Applying the age-old perspectives from blood product sterilization, researchers irradiated lungs in EVLP systems with ultraviolet C (UVC) light, which has been known for its germicidal properties [33, 34]. Similarly, another light-based sterilization technique called photodynamic therapy (PDT) uses methylene blue irradiated with red light [35]. As compared to standard EVLP, which focused simply on washing the virus away from the organ, PDT was the most effective in reducing HCV load. It cleared 98% of HCV-RNA from the perfusate and 91% from the lung tissue. The UVC group did not show any significant reduction as compared to controls [33, 36]. Despite reduced infectivity of the persistent RNA fragments noticed in *in vitro* analysis, UVC irradiation failed to prevent the development of viremia posttransplant in further trials [37]. Is it hypothesized that this difference arises because of the weaker penetrating power of UVC rays due to wavelength differences as compared to PDT [38]. Additionally, irradiated methylene blue provided better coverage because it could be injected into the vasculature [36].

The potential of EVLP for research and to evaluate and salvage initially rejected lungs is vast and the outcomes after using EVLP are comparable to standard lung transplantation. Multiple trials are demonstrating ingenious ways to utilize the technology clinically [27]. For example, researchers are administering targeted adenosine receptor 2B antagonists via EVLP to abolish its proinflammatory effects [39]. The use of EVLP as a platform for improving the utilization of donated lungs continues to increase.

Recently, Cypel et al. identified 10°C to be an optimal temperature for lung storage, allowing for preservation times of up to 24–36°C. Furthermore, they explored the concept of multiday lung preservation by pairing 10°C lung preservation with short cycles of EVLP in an animal model. For the first time, they were successful 3-days of lung preservation with exceptional immediate posttransplant graft function [40].

Loor et al., in the INSPIRE trial, sought to assess the safety and efficacy of normothermic portable EVLP using the OCS Lung device. It was the first prospective, multicenter, and randomized controlled study in EVLP for standard bilateral lung transplantation. The composite primary effectiveness endpoint of the trial was absence of PGD 3 within the first 72 hours after transplant and 30-day survival in the per-protocol population, with a 4% noninferiority margin [41]. The EXPAND trial was used to evaluate the efficacy of normothermic portable organ care system (OCS) lung perfusion and ventilation on donor lung use from extended-criteria donors and donors after circulatory death. OCS resulted in 87% of donor lung use for transplantation with excellent clinical outcomes [42]. A major challenge in lung transplantation is the need for ABO blood group matching. To address this challenge, Wang et al. used two enzymes, FpGalNAc deacetylase and FpGalactosaminidase, to convert blood group A lungs to blood group O lungs during *ex vivo* lung perfusion. The authors demonstrated successful removal of blood group A antigen with no overt changes in lung health. The authors showed reduced antibody and complement deposition, suggesting that this technique may reduce antibody-mediated injury *in vivo* [43].

6.1 Lung transportation

Conventional cold static preservation of donor's lungs leads to unpredictable lung tissue cooling as also the freezing and thawing cause irreversible cellular damage. The Paragonix LUNGguard donor preservation system provides a stable temperature between 4 and 8°C for extended preservation times. Hartwig et al. presented their initial report of a study comparing two methodologies of hypothermic storage: patients with donor lungs preserved by the LUNGguard and patients with donor lungs transported by conventional preservation methods (ice protocol) [44].

6.2 Intraoperative use of cardiopulmonary bypass (CPB) vs. ECMO for lung transplantation

The use of extracorporeal membrane oxygenation (ECMO) for intraoperative cardiopulmonary support has gained traction in recent years. There is growing experience with the preoperative use of ECMO as a bridge to a transplant in patients with refractory respiratory failure. Biscotti et al. compared differences in patient outcomes and operative parameters for extracorporeal membrane oxygenation (ECMO) versus cardiopulmonary bypass (CPB) in patients undergoing lung transplants. Intraoperatively, CPB group required more cell saver volume, FFP, platelets, and cryoprecipitate. The CPB group had higher rates of primary graft dysfunction at 24 and 72 hours. There were no differences in 30-day and 1-year survivals [45]. Hoetzenecker et al., from the Vienna lung transplant group reported their results of uniform central venoarterial ECMO in patients receiving bilateral lung transplantation. Their median time of mechanical ventilation was 29 hours, 90-day mortality was 3.1%, and 2-year survival was 86%. Thus, routine use of intraoperative ECMO resulted in excellent primary graft function and midterm outcomes in patients undergoing lung transplantation [46]. Magoulitis et al. in their meta-analysis of seven observational studies incorporating 785 patients showed that ECMO support lowered rate of primary graft dysfunction, bleeding, renal failure requiring dialysis, tracheostomy, intraoperative transfusions, intubation time, and hospital stay. However, no difference was reported between operative and ischemic time [47]. Recently, Halpern et al. in their study on patients with no or mild pulmonary hypertension, who underwent bilateral lung transplantation, reported that planned VA ECMO was associated with higher odds of textbook outcomes than planned off-pump support [48].

7. Advances in treatment of post-lung transplant complications

According to the OPTN annual report in 2020, 14.6% of lung transplant recipients developed acute rejection. 40% of recipients went on to develop bronchiolitis obliterans syndrome (BOS) by the fifth year after transplant, and 24% of recipients developed malignancy in the same period.

Chronic lung allograft dysfunction (CLAD) holds substantial weightage during the discussion of lung transplant because it is a major cause of mortality and morbidity following lung transplantation [49]. According to the ISHLT consensus report 2019, CLAD is a persistent > = 20% decline in FEV1 as compared to the recipient's posttransplant baseline [50]. Decreases in lung functions after three months posttransplant are also attributed to CLAD. Two prominent subtypes of CLAD are BOS

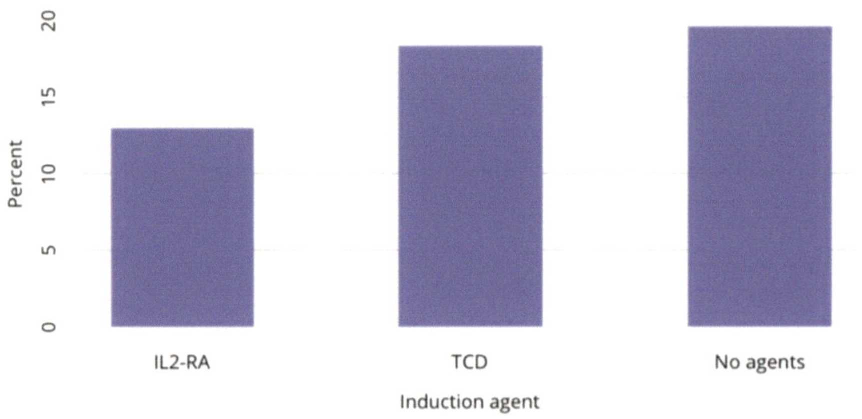

Figure 3.
Incidence of acute rejection by 1-year posttransplant among adult lung transplant recipients by induction agent, 2018–2019. Only the first reported rejection event is counted. Cumulative incidence is estimated using the Kaplan–Meier method. IL2-RA, interleukin-2 receptor agonist; TCD, T-cell depleting. (from OPTN/SRTR 2020 annual data report. HHS/HRSA).

(bronchiolitis obliterans syndrome) and RAS (restrictive allograft syndrome) [49]. Once BOS develops, the mortality rate varies from 25 to 55% [51, 52]. Risk factors of CLAD include autoimmunity, PGD, alloimmune rejections (e.g., acute cellular rejection, antibody-mediated rejection, and lymphocytic bronchiolitis), infections (viral, bacterial, and fungal), persistent bronchoalveolar lavage neutrophilia and pathological gastroesophageal reflux (**Figure 3**) [31].

Newer treatment modalities, such as extracorporeal photopheresis (which uses ultraviolet light to generate anti-inflammatory cytokines), liposomal cyclosporine, and anti-fibrotic agents, such as pirfenidone, are being assessed in the treatment of CLAD in trials.

8. Lung transplantation committee

Recently, a collaborative effort of transplant centers has led to formation of a committee. The lung transplantation committee of OPTN works regarding lung procurement, allocation, and transplantation, including medical, scientific, and ethical aspects. The goal of the committee's work is to develop evidence-based policies aimed at reducing waitlist mortality in lung transplant candidates, increasing lung utilization, improving access to lung transplantation, and improving the health outcomes of lung transplant recipients.

9. Lung microbiome

The characteristics of the lung microbiome, its influence on the human body and disease processes, and the techniques to alter the local microbiome, serve as a large reservoir of untapped knowledge. Studies have been constantly trying to understand the differences between the microbiome of a healthy lung and a diseased one. 16S rRNA sequencing studies have disclosed that the lung microbiome is derived majorly from the oropharynx, with prevotella, veillonella, and streptococcus spp. being the most frequent colonizers [53, 54]. Consequently, it has been postulated that disruption of the oropharyngeal microbiome will reflect in the lung and ultimately make it more susceptible to pathogen colonization [55]. It is also being hypothesized that a healthy lung microbiome is based on the property of the organisms to be transient, owing to the dynamicity attributed to breathing and microaspiration. The microbial ecosystem of the lung is maintained delicately by a balance between the entry and active clearance by the cells of the lung. When the mechanisms of clearance fail, the organisms become persistent and disease ensues. It remains to be elucidated as to whether dysbiosis is a cause or effect of the disease [56]. Conventional literature believed that certain disease processes or exposures had a singular effect on the host. Recent studies, while acknowledging its effect on the microbiome independently, go beyond this idea and hypothesize that even without external influences, the microbiome and the host continually modulate each other [57].

Researchers have analyzed the oropharyngeal microbial pattern in patients with end-stage lung diseases, before and after lung transplantation. While waiting for transplantation, it was found that oropharyngeal wash samples of patients with advanced lung diseases had an increased facultative organism dominant microbial burden. Aerobic bacteria were decreased, alongside an overall reduction in richness and diversity. The microbiome stabilized after transplantation briefly, tending toward healthy lung levels. Nevertheless, 6 months after transplantation, it reverted to the severe dysbiosis-like state that existed before transplantation in the diseased lung [55]. If dysbiosis at oral sites indeed precedes/causes dysbiosis in the lungs, then these observations remind us of the increased risk of infections due to pathogen colonization posttransplantation, adding to the problems caused by an immunosuppressed state.

Studies have been working toward establishing and elaborating on the relationship between the altered microbiome and the complications after lung transplant. The most worrisome ones are primary graft dysfunction (PGD), acute rejection (AR), and chronic lung allograft dysfunction (CLAD). Lungs that had enrichment of oral-type taxa, before procurement from the donor and immediately after reperfusion in the recipient, have been seen to develop PGD. Aspiration of these microbes is hypothesized to prime the allografts for PGD [58]. Similarly, it is also observed that higher bacterial load after transplant is correlated with the development of CLAD, although no particular taxa were implicated [59]. These discoveries are promising as the microbiome can prove to be a potentially modifiable risk factor.

It is well known that inflammatory episodes happen in the allograft after transplantation, despite adequate immunosuppression [60]. Long-term immunosuppression and antibiotic therapy posttransplantation may make the local ecosystem more permissive to the overgrowth of certain immunostimulatory bacteria, which otherwise would have been cleared by the host immunity and controlled by the healthy microbiome [61, 62].

Inflammation can also be triggered by imbalances in the levels of normal commensals, which means that it is not necessary that a pathogenic invasion occurs for a disease process to ensue. For example, the Prevotella community is a part of the normal lung microbiome and is generally considered less stimulatory, but its overrepresentation can cause tissue remodeling [63]. In lung transplant recipients, an association between the dominant bacteria and the type of immune reaction was observed. When the dysbiosis was firmicutes or proteobacteria dominant, pulmonary leukocytes expressed inflammatory genes; while pro-remodeling effects were displayed by a Bacteroidetes-dominant dysbiosis [63]. Similarly, in the case of pathogens, virulence does not necessarily equate with immunogenicity. S. Pneumoniae, which is the most common cause of community-acquired pneumonia, had a lower stimulatory effect on macrophages in comparison with S.aureus or P.aeruginosa [63]. Hyperammonemia syndrome (HS) is an uncommon but fatal disorder that can affect up to 4% of lung transplant recipients. It is imperative that patients with this syndrome should be screened for ureaplasma species and treated with the appropriate antibiotics for this infection [64].

10. Gut-lung axis

The effects of the gut microbiome on local and systemic immunity are well studied, and the documentation of its influence on the brain led to the coining of the term "gut-brain axis." Investigators are now trying to find out if such a relationship also exists between the microbiome of the gut and the lung. Several studies indicate that such "gut-lung axis" may indeed exist. For example, gut microbiome dysbiosis caused by antibiotic administration in the early years of life was seen to increase the risk of allergic airway disease [65]. Fecal microbiomes in patients with chronic obstructive pulmonary disease differed from healthy control subjects in terms of taxonomic microbial representation and their metabolites [66]. Murine models that were dietarily supplemented with short-chain fatty acids (SCFA) by adding acetate to their drinking water showed reduced inflammatory infiltrates in their lungs. Au contraire, those receiving a low-fiber diet had lower SCFAs in their circulation and higher airway reactivity [67].

It has been recently found in clinical and animal studies that derangement in the gut microbiome can impact outcomes related to allograft dysfunction after transplantation of the liver and small bowel [68, 69]. To understand whether gut microbiome can impact lung allograft rejection as well mice model studies were conducted. The donors as well as recipients were pretreated with oral antibiotic gavages to reduce microbial load. Those that were pretreated had reduced severity of rejection, while the majority of the controls showed moderate–severe lung allograft rejection. The Bacteroidetes to firmicutes ratio was increased in the gut microbiome of the mice who experienced milder rejection [70]. Previous studies have tried to establish a causal link between CD4+ T lymphocytes and chronic lung allograft rejection in animal models after lung transplantation [71]. This would mean that a depletion of CD4+ T cells would improve the outcomes related to allograft rejection. However, an emerging hypothesis suggests that a reduced dendritic cell activation may instead be the origin of the decreased generation of graft-reactive T cells [70].

Unlike the gut microbiome, where microbial sampling is relatively easier due to their presence in the feces, determining the ecosystem of the lung is complicated by factors like lower biomass, the possibility of contamination during sample collection, interference by environmental factors, and the lack of knowledge about the fungal and viral component of the microbiome. Researchers have been citing the possibility of a metagenomic dark matter due to the presence of a large proportion of unidentified sequences arising during virome studies. This may indicate that we may come across undiscovered species of viruses in the future [72]. For example, recently, metagenomic sequencing from the respiratory tract of healthy as well as sick subjects led to the discovery of a new family of DNA viruses called redondoviridae [73].

More techniques are needed to profile the lung microbiome more accurately, to understand how the interactions affect the host, to establish causality between dysbiosis and specific disease processes, and to observe the resolution of symptoms after the reestablishment of the original microbiome. It would be interesting to see how therapeutic alteration of the microbiome can impact not only the outcomes of lung transplantation but also chronic disease processes in general. Trials are now being proposed to observe the effect of therapies like probiotic administration and fecal microbiota transplantation in the context of respiratory diseases [74]. If endotypes can be targeted specifically, it could open up multiple avenues tailored to deliver a personalized benefit [75]. The prospects of lung microbiome research are certainly promising but long-term studies will be necessary to ascertain the benefits quantitatively.

11. Bioengineering

Bioengineered lungs could change the landscape of lung transplantation as they counter the challenges posed by the long waitlist [76]. These techniques revolve around harvesting a lung sample and decellularizing it. The scaffold (acellular or artificial or hybrid) is then recellularized with stem or differentiated cells [77]. The matured and functional organ is then implanted into the host. EVLP systems serve as a good conduit to allow the maturation of the engineered graft [76, 78–80]. The fusion of current methods with emerging single-cell technologies and advanced 3D printing modalities could pave way for newer developments [81]. Substantial efforts are necessary to refine the existing engineering techniques and to convert preclinical studies to clinical trials in order to manifest this idea as a utilitarian alternative [76]. The idea of the bioengineered lung which appeared like utopian fiction decades ago could soon become reality [81].

12. Recent advances in heart transplantation

As a testament to improved survival statistics, heart transplant recipients have had an improved prognosis over the years. Since 2015, adult long-term mortality rates have witnessed a downward trend. Similarly, pretransplant mortality rates have also declined since 2009 [2]. However, this scenario was complicated by the COVID-19 pandemic, where we saw an increase in the 6-month and 1-year mortality rates during the first year of the pandemic. Pretransplant mortality also slightly increased in 2020 (**Figure 4**) [2]. Heart transplant candidates have notable changes in demographic patterns over the years. Candidates over 65 years of age have increased from 11.9% in 2009 to 15.9% in 2020. The prevalence of obesity has increased among heart transplant candidates. As of 2020, more than 40% of candidates have a BMI equal to or more than 30 kg/m2 [2]. Cardiomyopathy remains the most common indication for an adult heart transplant, while congenital heart disease remains the leading diagnosis in the pediatric age group. Notably, candidates receiving transplantation for a diagnosis of coronary artery disease have declined [2]. Continued efforts of the entire healthcare system have helped in improving transplant-related outcomes despite the current COVID-19 pandemic. Fewer candidates have been removed from the waitlist because of death or being too sick to receive transplants as compared to 2018 [2]. The number of multiple organ transplants has also increased, which is appreciated in heart-kidney transplants, while heart-lung transplants have remained stable [2]. In 2020, despite there being lesser new listings for heart transplants, the eventual number of heart transplants performed increased [2].

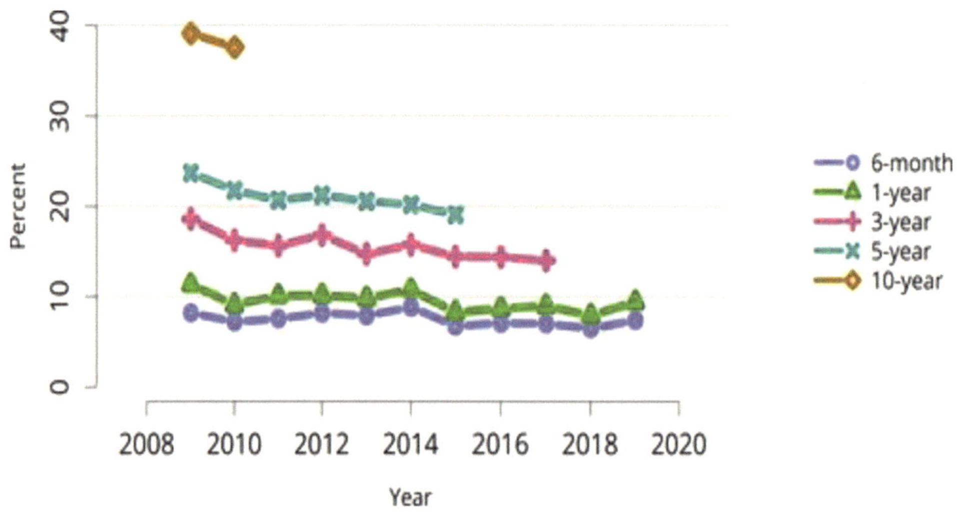

Figure 4.
Patient death among adult heart transplant recipients. All adult recipients of deceased donor hearts, including multi-organ transplants (from OPTN/SRTR 2020 annual data report. HHS/HRSA).

The number of deceased heart donors continues to increase. The discard rate of recovered organs remains extremely low at 1%, despite a slight rise in 2020. An upward trend is noted in the proportion of IRDs [2]. In the case of heart transplants, the use of mechanical circulatory support (MCS) as a bridge to transplant has dramatically increased over the years. In 2020, 36.4% of candidates had ventricular assist devices (VAD) at listing. This number was just 16.4% in 2010 [2].

To address the issue of waitlist mortality, the year 2018 witnessed new heart allocation criteria, as approved by the united network for organ sharing (UNOS). These criteria prioritized the sickest patients. The older 3-tier system (status 1A, 1B, and 2) was changed to a 6-tier one (status 1–6) [82]. Stable patients supported by LVAD were ranked lower (status 4) as compared to those receiving VA-ECMO and IABP, status 1 and 2, respectively [83].

Traditionally, for prolonged support, ventricular assist devices needed to be placed after securing surgical access. This was especially true when candidates were being bridged to transplant [84]. Recently, more research is being done on assist devices that can be implanted percutaneously. After the UNOS heart allocation policy change, the use of percutaneous devices like Impella jumped from 1% in 2015 to 4% in 2019 among transplant patients [85]. Impella is a catheter-based ventricular assist device for unloading the left ventricle and consequently increasing cardiac output. It was initially used to support patients with cardiogenic shock after acute myocardial infarction [86]. Due to its relative ease of insertion, it is now being considered as an alternative to support candidates waiting for a heart transplant. As compared to recipients who did not receive circulatory support, patients bridged to transplant using Impella 5.0/5.5 showed a similar 30-day and 6-month mortality [84, 87, 88].

13. Donation after circulatory death, organ care system, and normothermic regional perfusion

The standard cold ice transport of donor's hearts results in unpredictable myocardial cooling leading to irreversible suppression of diastolic function and protein denaturation. The recently introduced Paragonix SherpaPak Cardiac Transport System incorporates a novel nested canister system in concert with proprietary thermal cooling to provide physical and thermal protection for donor's hearts. Results of 1-year transplant survival analysis of GAURDIAN registry showed that despite longer ischemic times and higher proportions of temporary MCS devices, numerically higher 1-year survival was seen in the cohort with sherapak usage [89]. Dhittal et al. pioneered the technique of DCD heart procurement. Their technique allows for rapid decompression of the systemic venous system and subsequent cardioplegia administration. Following infusion of supplemented cardioplegia, the heart is explanted first and instrumented onto the portable extracorporeal TransMedics organ care system (OCS), where its viability and suitability for transplantation can be assessed [90].

13.1 Organ care system

An OCS heart is a portable extracorporeal heart perfusion and monitoring system. The aorta is connected to the aortic line, the pulmonary artery is connected to the pulmonary artery line (PA line), the left atrium is opened, and the left ventricle is vented via a left ventricle vent. The superior and inferior vena cava are ligated. Blood from the PA line and LV vent goes to the reservoir and is pumped to the gas exchanger where it is oxygenated, passed through a warmer, and returned to the heart through the aortic line. It allows continuous monitoring of aortic pressure, lactate level, and coronary blood flow of the graft. The advantages of OCS are:

1. It enables the donor heart to be transported for long distances, thereby increasing the donor pool.

2. The aortic perfusion on the OCS system can act as a surrogate to diagnose significant coronary artery disease in the donor's heart.

3. Increasing the pool of marginal donor hearts (hearts with left ventricular hypertrophy, EF 40–50%, downtime more than 20 minutes, and donor age > 55 years).

In the EXPAND trial, out of 93 such marginal hearts, 75 hearts were transplanted (81% utilization rate). The mean cross-clamp time and OCS perfusion time were 381 minutes and 279 minutes, respectively. In this study, the 30-day survival was 95%, the incidence of severe primary graft dysfunction within 24 hours of transplant was 11%, and the overall and graft survival at 24 months was 82% and 95%, respectively.

4. It provides a platform to assess DCD hearts prior to implantation.

However, the present limitation of the OCS is the additional cost of resources and personnel required for its application as well as its transportation is more complicated [91].

13.2 Normothermic regional perfusion

The alternate method of DCD heart procurement is normothermic regional perfusion (NRP) wherein VA-ECMO is utilized (by cannulating aorta and right atrium) to maintain the thoracic organ perfusion to allow them to recover warm ischemia. The advantages of NRP are:

1. It restores heart function by reducing myocardial injury.

2. Reduces time spent by the organ in warm ischemia.

3. Allows visual assessment of heart and other organs prior to procurement.

The utilization of NRP for DCD requires significant resources and coordination between the donor hospital, procurement teams, and organ procurement organizations [92].

14. Post-heart transplant rejection surveillance

Between 2018 and 2019, 23.6% of recipients of heart transplants suffered from acute rejection in one year [2]. Even though the gold standard for posttransplant rejection surveillance is an endomyocardial biopsy, there have been exciting developments in the past decade in molecular noninvasive diagnostic surveillance. Such novel molecular techniques have the capacity to facilitate early diagnosis, improve the accuracy of diagnosis and decrease the frequency of invasive interventions for the diagnosis of allograft rejection [93].

14.1 Microarray technology

This technology examines endomyocardial biopsy samples at a molecular level to diagnose acute cellular rejection (ACR) as well as antibody-mediated rejection (AMR) [94]. Molecules called rejection associated transcripts (RAT) are identified to assess mRNA expression. Probabilities of developing ACR and AMR are then deduced. This technique was first implemented in patients who underwent kidney transplants. Halloran et al. later found out that similar RAT expression was observed in heart biopsy specimens, thus leading to the extrapolation of the idea in heart transplantation. This technique aims to tackle the main drawback of traditional histopathologic biopsies, which is interobserver variability in reporting findings [93, 95].

Currently, microarray technology is employed by the molecular microscope diagnostic system, which does an unsupervised archetypal analysis and predicts a normal, ACR, AMR, or injury pattern based on the assignment of scores [95]. This technology has been found to be effective in predicting molecular rejection [96]. The utility of intragraft mRNA transcripts as an addendum to the histopathology reports of endomyocardial biopsies can pave way for a newer modus operandi in diagnosing cardiac transplant rejection [93].

14.2 Gene expression profiling

Gene expression profiling (GEP) is done using peripheral blood leukocytes. It is done after 55 days posttransplant and has a high negative predictive value for moderate to severe rejection [93, 97]. Thus, it is used as an effective screening tool in stable posttransplant patients for diagnosis of rejection [93]. Allomap (CareDx) is the presently utilized gene expression profiling test in the clinical domain, which assigns a score of 0–40. A watershed score of > = 34 signals a higher probability of ACR [93, 98]. According to both IMAGE and E-IMAGE (early-IMAGE) clinical trials, GEP was found non-inferior to routine endomyocardial biopsy surveillance techniques, thus demonstrating similar clinical composite outcomes and rates of rejection [99, 100]. However, its use is limited only to the detection of ACR. Additionally, it also harbors a poor positive predictive value [93]. The CARGO-II trial proposed that a score less than 34 can imply a low risk of rejection [101]. Allomap can be utilized to time an early steroid weaning in patients with a lower risk of rejection [93].

14.3 Donor-derived cell-free DNA

This noninvasive modality of investigation is based on the cell death of the graft tissue, which releases donor-derived cell-free DNA (dd cfDNA) in the recipient's blood. The percentage of donor-derived cell-free DNA is titrated against the total cell-free DNA in the recipient's blood, detecting both ACR and AMR. It has also been found that dd cfDNA leads to earlier detection of acute rejection in asymptomatic patients compared to endomyocardial biopsy. The figure given below depicts the correlation between the percentage of dd cfDNA with ACR, AMR, and echocardiographic findings [93].

A study was conducted in Canada during the global COVID-19 pandemic utilizing noninvasive surveillance techniques for heart transplant rejection, thus ensuring minimal hospital exposure to patients. The study used cell-free DNA and gene expression profiling as a substitute for the invasive endomyocardial biopsy. The results were then harnessed for personalized titration of immunosuppressive therapy in patients. Noninvasive rejection surveillance was associated with the ability to lower immunosuppression, increase satisfaction, and reduce anxiety in HT recipients, minimizing exposure for patients and providers during a global pandemic [102].

15. Xenotransplantation

Xenotransplantation could act as a bridge to allotransplantation to tide over the crisis posed by the ever-growing waitlist. Recent developments have been in the domain of genetically engineered pigs functioning as donors for human recipients. Naturally occurring human antibodies commonly target 3 carbohydrate antigens in pigs among which galactose-a1,3-galactose is postulated to be particularly important. Removal of galactose-a1,3-galactose as antigen from pig yields a GTKO (*alpha* 1,3-galactosyltransferase knockout) pig. With the advent of novel gene editing techniques, double and triple-knockout pigs, engineered after the elimination of multiple carbohydrate coding genes were created.

Relatively species-specific complement pathway regulatory proteins (CPRP) like CD55, CD59, and CD56 attenuated complement-mediated injury and improved graft survival in various nonhuman primate models. These were introduced into the genome of pigs. Despite the addition of hCPRP (human complement pathway regulatory proteins) modification in GTKO pigs; the grafts were affected by microvascular thrombosis. This was probably due to a disharmony of thromboregulatory molecules like pig thrombomodulin and pig endothelial protein C receptor, which could be of a lower antithrombotic efficacy than their human counterparts. CD47 functions as a self-recognition marker in humans, which serves to inhibit phagocytosis. The Introduction of CD47 in the genome of pigs has shown better outcomes. Recently on January 7, 2022, the University of Maryland performed the first clinical heart xenotransplantation in a 57-year-old man, from a genetically engineered pig having 10 genetic modifications. He lived with a reasonable heart function for 2 months following the transplant but went on to develop graft dysfunction and ultimately, death. This event has however infused euphoria in the field of xenotransplantation and thoracic organ transplant academia. Similarly, in June/July 2022, Moazami et al. from New York University Langone successfully performed two further xenotransplants (pig hearts into humans) utilizing 10 genetic modifications, including four porcine gene "knockouts" to prevent rejection and abnormal organ growth as well as six human transgenes ("knock-ins") to promote expression of proteins that regulate important biologic pathways that can be disrupted by incompatibilities between pigs and humans.

Conflict of interest

The authors have nothing to disclose.

Abbreviations

COPD	chronic obstructive pulmonary disease
IIP	idiopathic interstitial pneumonia

CF	cystic fibrosis
CFTR	cystic fibrosis transmembrane conductance regulator
BMI	body mass index
ECMO	extracorporeal membrane oxygenation
OPTN	organ procurement & transplantation network
IRD	increased risk donor
HIV	human immunodeficiency virus
HBV	Hepatitis B virus
HCV	Hepatitis C virus
ODD	overdose death donor
TDD	trauma death donor
MDD	medical death donor
DAA	direct acting antivirals
NAT	nucleic acid testing
HOPE	HIV organ policy equity
HAART	highly active antiretroviral therapy
PLWH	people living with HIV
	HIV D+/R + transplant from HIV+ donor to HIV+ recipient.
	HIV D−/R + transplant from HIV- donor to HIV+ recipient.
EVLP	*ex vivo* lung perfusion
PGD	primary graft dysfunction
UVC	ultraviolet C
PDT	photodynamic therapy
ISHLT	international society for heart and lung transplants
CLAD	chronic lung allograft dysfunction
BOS	bronchiolitis obliterans syndrome
RAS	restrictive allograft syndrome
rRNA	ribosomal ribonucleic acid
AR	acute rejection
SCFA	short-chain fatty acids
	CD4+ T lymphocytes.
DNA	deoxyribonucleic acid
MCS	mechanical circulatory support
VAD	ventricular assist device
UNOS	united network for organ sharing
IABP	intra-aortic balloon pump
VA-ECMO	veno-arterial extracorporeal membrane oxygenation
ACR	acute cellular rejection
AMR	antibody-mediated rejection
RAT	rejection-associated transcripts
mRNA	messenger ribonucleic acid
GEP	gene expression profiling
IMAGE Trial	invasive monitoring attenuation through gene expression trial
E-IMAGE Trial	early-invasive monitoring attenuation through gene expression trial
CARGO-II Trial	cardiac allograft rejection gene expression observational trial -II
CfDNA	cell-free DNA
Dd cfDNA	donor-derived cell-free DNA
CPRP	complement pathway regulatory proteins
hCPRP	human complement pathway regulatory proteins
GTKO	alpha 1,3-galactosyltransferase knockout

WLST	withdrawal of life-sustaining treatment
OCS	organ care system
NRP	normothermic regional perfusion
DCD	donation after circulatory death

Author details

Akshay Kumar[1*], Sania Thite[2], Varad Wazarkar[2], Kamal Ayyat[1,3], Jesus Gomez Abraham[4] and Suresh Keshavamurthy[5]

1 Department of Thoracic and Cardiothoracic Surgery, Heart, Vascular and Thoracic Institute, Cleveland Clinic, Cleveland, Ohio, United States

2 Lokmanya Tilak Municipal Medical College, Mumbai, India

3 Department of Inflammation and Immunity, Lerner Research Institute, Cleveland Clinic, Cleveland, Ohio, United States

4 Department of Cardiothoracic Surgery, Newark Beth Israel Medical Center, Newark, New Jersey

5 Division of Cardiothoracic Surgery, Surgical Director Lung Transplantation, University of Kentucky College of Medicine, Kentucky, United States

*Address all correspondence to: drakshay82@gmail.com

References

[1] International Society for Heart and Lung Transplantation. Adult and pediatric lung transplants: Number of transplants by year and procedure type. JHLT. 2019;**38**(10):1015-1066

[2] Organ Procurement and Transplantation Network (OPTN) and Scientific Registry of Transplant Recipients (SRTR). OPTN/SRTR 2020 Annual Data Report. Rockville, MD: Department of Health and Human Services, Health Resources and Services Administration; 2022

[3] Bock MJ, Vaughn GR, Chau P, Berumen JA, Nigro JJ, et al. Organ transplantation using COVID-19-positive deceased donors. American Journal of Transplantation. 2022;**22**(9):2203-2216. DOI: 10.1111/ajt.17145

[4] Eichenberger EM, Coniglio AC, Milano C, Schroder J, Bryner BS, et al. Transplanting thoracic COVID-19 positive donors: An institutional protocol and report of the first 14 cases. The Journal of Heart and Lung Transplantation. 2022;**41**(10):1376-1381. DOI: 10.1016/j.healun.2022.06.018

[5] International Society for Heart and Lung Transplantation. Adult lung transplants: Recipient characteristics. JHLT. 2021;**40**(10):1023-1072

[6] International Society for Heart and Lung Transplantation. Adult Lung Transplants: Diagnoses. JHLT. 2019;**38**(10):1015-1066

[7] Keshavamurthy S, Rodgers-Fischl P. Donation after circulatory death (DCD)-lung procurement. Indian Journal of Thoracic Cardiovascular Surgery. 2021;**37**(Suppl 3):425-432. DOI: 10.1007/s12055-021-01156-7

[8] Healey A, Watanabe Y, Mills C, Stoncius M, Lavery S, et al. Initial lung transplantation experience with uncontrolled donation after cardiac death in North America. American Journal of Transplantation. 2020;**20**(6):1574-1581. DOI: 10.1111/ajt.15795

[9] Leard LE, Holm AM, Valapour M, Glanville AR, Attawar S, et al. Consensus document for the selection of lung transplant candidates: An update from the International Society for Heart and Lung Transplantation. The Journal of Heart and Lung Transplantation. 2021;**40**(11):1349-1379. DOI: 10.1016/j.healun.2021.07.005

[10] Seem DL, Lee I, Umscheid CA, Kuehnert MJ. United States Public Health Service. PHS guideline for reducing human immunodeficiency virus, hepatitis B virus, and hepatitis C virus transmission through organ transplantation. Public Health Reports. 2013;**128**(4):247-343. DOI: 10.1177/003335491312800403

[11] Durand CM, Bowring MG, Thomas AG, Kucirka LM, Massie AB, et al. The drug overdose epidemic and deceased-donor transplantation in the United States: A National Registry Study. Annals of Internal Medicine. 2018;**168**(10):702-711. DOI: 10.7326/M17-2451

[12] Sapiano MRP, Jones JM, Bowman J, Levi ME, Basavaraju SV. Impact of US public health service increased risk deceased donor designation on organ utilization. American Journal of Transplantation. 2019;**19**(9):2560-2569. DOI: 10.1111/ajt.15388

[13] Woolley AE, Piechura LM, Goldberg HJ, Singh SK, Coppolino A, et al. The impact of hepatitis C viremic donor lung allograft characteristics on

post-transplantation outcomes. Annals of Cardiothoracic Surgery. 2020;**9**(1):42-48. DOI: 10.21037/acs.2020.01.03

[14] Feld JJ, Cypel M, Kumar D, Dahari H, Pinto Ribeiro RV, et al. Short-course, direct-acting antivirals and ezetimibe to prevent HCV infection in recipients of organs from HCV-infected donors: A phase 3, single-Centre, open-label study. The Lancet Gastroenterology & Hepatology. 2020;**5**(7):649-657. DOI: 10.1016/S2468-1253(20)30081-9

[15] Kwong AJ, Wall A, Melcher M, Wang U, Ahmed A, et al. Liver transplantation for hepatitis C virus (HCV) non-viremic recipients with HCV viremic donors. American Journal of Transplantation. 2019;**19**(5):1380-1387. DOI: 10.1111/ajt.15162

[16] Suryaprasad A, Basavaraju SV, Hocevar SN, Theodoropoulos N, Zuckerman RA, et al. Organ transplantation hepatitis C investigation team. Transmission of hepatitis C virus from organ donors despite nucleic acid test screening. American Journal of Transplantation. 2015;**15**(7):1827-1835. DOI: 10.1111/ajt.13283

[17] Orens JB, Estenne M, Arcasoy S, Conte JV, Corris P, et al. Pulmonary scientific Council of the International Society for heart and lung transplantation. International guidelines for the selection of lung transplant candidates: 2006 update--a consensus report from the pulmonary scientific Council of the International Society for heart and lung transplantation. The Journal of Heart and Lung Transplantation. 2006;**25**(7):745-755. DOI: 10.1016/j.healun.2006.03.011

[18] Rouzaud C et al. Lung transplantation in HIV patients. The Journal of Heart and Lung Transplantation. 2022;**41**(4):S531-S532

[19] Koval CE, Farr M, Krisl J, Haidar G, Pereira MR, et al. Heart or lung transplant outcomes in HIV-infected recipients. The Journal of Heart and Lung Transplantation. 2019;**38**(12):1296-1305. DOI: 10.1016/j.healun.2019.09.011

[20] Klitenic SB, Levan ML, Van Pilsum Rasmussen SE, Durand CM. Science over stigma: Lessons and future direction of HIV-to-HIV transplantation. Current Transplantion Reports. 2021;**8**(4):314-323. DOI: 10.1007/s40472-021-00345-y

[21] Redd AD, Quinn TC, Tobian AA. Frequency and implications of HIV superinfection. The Lancet Infectious Diseases. 2013;**13**(7):622-628. DOI: 10.1016/S1473-3099(13)70066-5

[22] Stock PG, Barin B, Murphy B, Hanto D, Diego JM, et al. Outcomes of kidney transplantation in HIV-infected recipients. The New England Journal of Medicine. 2010;**363**(21):2004-2014. DOI: 10.1056/NEJMoa1001197

[23] Canaud G, Dejucq-Rainsford N, Avettand-Fenoël V, Viard JP, Anglicheau D, et al. The kidney as a reservoir for HIV-1 after renal transplantation. Journal of American Society of Nephrology. 2014;**25**(2):407-419. DOI: 10.1681/ASN.2013050564

[24] Durand CM, Zhang W, Brown DM, Yu S, Desai N, et al. HOPE in action investigators. A prospective multicenter pilot study of HIV-positive deceased donor to HIV-positive recipient kidney transplantation: HOPE in action. American Journal of Transplantation. 2021;**21**(5):1754-1764. DOI: 10.1111/ajt.16205

[25] Predmore Z, Doby B, Bozzi DG, Durand C, Segev D, et al. Barriers experienced by organ procurement organizations in implementing the HOPE act and HIV-positive organan

donation. AIDS Care. 2021;**34**:1-7. DOI: 10.1080/09540121.2021.1945999

[26] Chan PG, Kumar A, Subramaniam K, Sanchez PG. Ex vivo lung perfusion: A review of research and clinical practices. Seminars in Cardiothoracic and Vascular Anesthesia. 2020;**24**(1):34-44. DOI: 10.1177/1089253220905147

[27] Okamoto T, Niikawa H, Ayyat K, et al. Machine perfusion of lungs. Current Transplant Report. 2019;**6**:251-264. DOI: 10.1007/s40472-019-00258-x

[28] Ayyat KS, Okamoto T, Niikawa H, Sakanoue I, Dugar S, et al. A CLUE for better assessment of donor lungs: Novel technique in clinical ex vivo lung perfusion. The Journal of Heart and Lung Transplantation. 2020;**39**(11):1220-1227. DOI: 10.1016/j.healun.2020.07.013

[29] Porteous MK, Diamond JM, Christie JD. Primary graft dysfunction: Lessons learned about the first 72h after lung transplantation. Current Opinion in Organ Transplantation. 2015;**20**(5):506-514. DOI: 10.1097/MOT.0000000000000232

[30] Cypel M, Yeung JC, Liu M, Anraku M, Chen F, et al. Normothermic ex vivo lung perfusion in clinical lung transplantation. The New England Journal of Medicine. 2011;**364**(15):1431-1440. DOI: 10.1056/NEJMoa1014597

[31] Meyer KC. Recent advances in lung transplantation. F1000Res. 2018;7:F1000. DOI: 10.12688/f1000research.15393.1

[32] Nakajima D, Cypel M, Bonato R, Machuca TN, Iskender I, et al. Ex vivo perfusion treatment of infection in human donor lungs. American Journal of Transplantation. 2016;**16**(4):1229-1237. DOI: 10.1111/ajt.13562

[33] Galasso M, Feld JJ, Watanabe Y, Pipkin M, Summers C, et al. Inactivating hepatitis C virus in donor lungs using light therapies during normothermic ex vivo lung perfusion. Nature Communications. 2019;**10**(1):481. DOI: 10.1038/s41467-018-08261-z

[34] Mohr H, Steil L, Gravemann U, Thiele T, Hammer E, et al. A novel approach to pathogen reduction in platelet concentrates using short-wave ultraviolet light. Transfusion. 2009;**49**(12):2612-2624. DOI: 10.1111/j.1537-2995.2009.02334.x

[35] Müller-Breitkreutz K, Mohr H. Hepatitis C and human immunodeficiency virus RNA degradation by methylene blue/light treatment of human plasma. Journal of Medical Virology. 1998;**56**(3):239-245. DOI: 10.1002/(sici)1096-9071(199811)56:3<239::aid-jmv11>3.0.co;2-9

[36] Ribeiro RVP, Ali A, Cypel M. Ex vivo perfusion in lung transplantation and removal of HCV: The next level. Transplant International. 2020;**33**(12):1589-1596. DOI: 10.1111/tri.13730

[37] Cypel M, Feld JJ, Galasso M, Pinto Ribeiro RV, Marks N, et al. Prevention of viral transmission during lung transplantation with hepatitis C-viraemic donors: An open-label, single-Centre, pilot trial. The Lancet Respiratory Medicine. 2020;**8**(2):192-201. DOI: 10.1016/S2213-2600(19)30268-1

[38] Wang HW, Zhu TC, Putt ME, Solonenko M, Metz J, et al. Broadband reflectance measurements of light penetration, blood oxygenation, hemoglobin concentration, and drug concentration in human intraperitoneal tissues before and after photodynamic therapy. Journal of Biomedical Optics. 2005;**10**(1):14004. DOI: 10.1117/1.1854679

[39] Huerter ME, Sharma AK, Zhao Y, Charles EJ, Kron IL, et al. Attenuation of

pulmonary ischemia-reperfusion injury by adenosine A2B receptor antagonism. The Annals of Thoracic Surgery. 2016;**102**(2):385-393. DOI: 10.1016/j.athoracsur.2016.02.060

[40] Ali A, Nykanen AI, Beroncal E, Brambate E, Mariscal A, et al. Successful 3-day lung preservation using a cyclic normothermic ex vivo lung perfusion strategy. eBioMedicine. 2022;**83**:104210. DOI: 10.1016/j.ebiom.2022.104210

[41] Loor G, Parulekar A, Smith M. Evaluation of the INSPIRE trial and its implications for lung transplantation with normothermic portable ex vivo lung perfusion. The Journal of Thoracic and Cardiovascular Surgery. 2019;**158**(4):1259-1263. DOI: 10.1016/j.jtcvs.2019.02.139

[42] Loor G, Warnecke G, Villavicencio MA, Smith MA, Kukreja J, et al. Portable normothermic ex-vivo lung perfusion, ventilation, and functional assessment with the organ care system on donor lung use for transplantation from extended-criteria donors (EXPAND): A single-arm, pivotal trial. The Lancet Respiratory Medicine. 2019;7(11):975-984. DOI: 10.1016/S2213-2600(19)30200-0

[43] Wang A, Ribeiro RVP, Ali A, Brambate E, Abdelnour-Berchtold E, et al. Ex vivo enzymatic treatment converts blood type a donor lungs into universal blood type lungs. Science Translational Medicine. 2022;**14**(632):eabm7190. DOI: 10.1126/scitranslmed.abm7190

[44] Hartwig M, Bush E, Langer N, Haney J. Report of the GUARDIAN-LUNG registry: An analysis of advanced hypothermic preservation on lung transplantation. The Journal of Heart and Lung Transplantation. 2022;**41**(4):S37. DOI: 10.1016/j.healun.2022.01.084

[45] Biscotti M, Yang J, Sonett J, Bacchetta M. Comparison of extracorporeal membrane oxygenation versus cardiopulmonary bypass for lung transplantation. The Journal of Thoracic and Cardiovascular Surgery. 2014;**148**(5):2410-2415. DOI: 10.1016/j.jtcvs.2014.07.061

[46] Hoetzenecker K, Benazzo A, Stork T, Sinn K, Schwarz S, et al. Vienna lung transplant group. Bilateral lung transplantation on intraoperative extracorporeal membrane oxygenator: An observational study. The Journal of Thoracic and Cardiovascular Surgery. 2020;**160**(1):320-327.e1. DOI: 10.1016/j.jtcvs.2019.10.155

[47] Magouliotis DE, Tasiopoulou VS, Svokos AA, Svokos KA, Zacharoulis D. Extracorporeal membrane oxygenation versus cardiopulmonary bypass during lung transplantation: A meta-analysis. General Thoracic and Cardiovascular Surgery. 2018;**66**(1):38-47. DOI: 10.1007/s11748-017-0836-3

[48] Halpern SE, Wright MC, Madsen G, Chow B, Harris CS, Haney JC, et al. Textbook outcome in lung transplantation: Planned venoarterial extracorporeal membrane oxygenation versus off-pump support for patients without pulmonary hypertension. The Journal of Heart and Lung Transplantation. 2022;**41**(11):1628-1637. DOI: 10.1016/j.healun.2022.07.015

[49] Verleden GM, Glanville AR, Lease ED, Fisher AJ, Calabrese F, et al. Chronic lung allograft dysfunction: Definition, diagnostic criteria, and approaches to treatment-a consensus report from the pulmonary council of the ISHLT. The Journal of Heart and Lung Transplantation. 2019;**38**(5):493-503. DOI: 10.1016/j.healun.2019.03.009

[50] Glanville AR, Verleden GM, Todd JL, Benden C, Calabrese F, et al.

Chronic lung allograft dysfunction: Definition and update of restrictive allograft syndrome-a consensus report from the pulmonary council of the ISHLT. The Journal of Heart and Lung Transplantation. 2019;**38**(5):483-492. DOI: 10.1016/j.healun.2019.03.008

[51] Burton CM, Carlsen J, Mortensen J, Andersen CB, Milman N, et al. Long-term survival after lung transplantation depends on development and severity of bronchiolitis obliterans syndrome. The Journal of Heart and Lung Transplantation. 2007;**26**(7):681-686. DOI: 10.1016/j.healun.2007.04.004

[52] Sato M, Ohmori-Matsuda K, Saito T, Matsuda Y, Hwang DM, et al. Time-dependent changes in the risk of death in pure bronchiolitis obliterans syndrome (BOS). The Journal of Heart and Lung Transplantation. 2013;**32**(5):484-491. DOI: 10.1016/j.healun.2013.01.1054

[53] Moffatt MF, Cookson WO. The lung microbiome in health and disease. Clinical Medicine (London, England). 2017;**17**(6):525-529. DOI: 10.7861/clinmedicine.17-6-525

[54] Dickson RP, Erb-Downward JR, Freeman CM, McCloskey L, Falkowski NR, et al. Bacterial topography of the healthy human lower respiratory tract. MBio. 2017;**8**(1):e02287-e02216. DOI: 10.1128/mBio.02287-16

[55] Simon-Soro A, Sohn MB, McGinniss JE, Imai I, Brown MC, et al. Upper respiratory Dysbiosis with a facultative-dominated ecotype in advanced lung disease and dynamic change after lung transplant. Annals of the American Thoracic Society. 2019;**16**(11):1383-1391. DOI: 10.1513/AnnalsATS.201904-299OC

[56] Budden KF, Gellatly SL, Wood DL, Cooper MA, Morrison M, et al. Emerging pathogenic links between microbiota and the gut-lung axis. Nature Reviews. Microbiology. 2017;**15**(1):55-63. DOI: 10.1038/nrmicro.2016.142

[57] Dickson RP. The lung microbiome and ARDS. It is time to broaden the model. American Journal of Respiratory and Critical Care Medicine. 2018;**197**(5):549-551. DOI: 10.1164/rccm.201710-2096ED

[58] McGinniss JE, Whiteside SA, Deek RA, Simon-Soro A, Graham-Wooten J, et al. The lung allograft microbiome associates with pepsin, inflammation, and primary graft dysfunction. American Journal of Respiratory and Critical Care Medicine. 2022. DOI: 10.1164/rccm.202112-2786OC

[59] Combs MP, Wheeler DS, Luth JE, Falkowski NR, Walker NM, et al. Lung microbiota predict chronic rejection in healthy lung transplant recipients: A prospective cohort study. The Lancet Respiratory Medicine. 2021;**9**(6):601-612. DOI: 10.1016/S2213-2600(20)30405-7

[60] Nakajima T, Palchevsky V, Perkins DL, Belperio JA, Finn PW. Lung transplantation: Infection, inflammation, and the microbiome. Seminars in Immunopathology. 2011;**33**(2):135-156. DOI: 10.1007/s00281-011-0249-9

[61] Charlson ES, Diamond JM, Bittinger K, Fitzgerald AS, Yadav A, et al. Lung-enriched organisms and aberrant bacterial and fungal respiratory microbiota after lung transplant. American Journal of Respiratory and Critical Care Medicine. 2012;**186**(6):536-545. DOI: 10.1164/rccm.201204-0693OC

[62] Borewicz K, Pragman AA, Kim HB, Hertz M, Wendt C, et al. Longitudinal analysis of the lung microbiome in lung transplantation. FEMS Microbiology Letters. 2013;**339**(1):57-65. DOI: 10.1111/1574-6968.12053

[63] Bernasconi E, Pattaroni C, Koutsokera A, Pison C, Kessler R, et al. Airway microbiota determines innate cell inflammatory or tissue remodeling profiles in lung transplantation. American Journal of Respiratory and Critical Care Medicine. 2016;**194**(10):1252-1263. DOI: 10.1164/rccm.201512-2424OC

[64] Kumar A, Advani S, Asim K, Mohamed MA, Wani F, et al. Hyperammonemia in lung transplant patients and its management: A review. Indian Journal of Thoracic Cardiovascular Surgery. 2022;**38**(Suppl 2):335-346. DOI: 10.1007/s12055-021-01319-6

[65] Russell SL, Gold MJ, Hartmann M, Willing BP, Thorson L, et al. Early life antibiotic-driven changes in microbiota enhance susceptibility to allergic asthma. EMBO Reports. 2012;**13**(5):440-447. DOI: 10.1038/embor.2012.32

[66] Bowerman KL, Rehman SF, Vaughan A, Lachner N, Budden KF, et al. Disease-associated gut microbiome and metabolome changes in patients with chronic obstructive pulmonary disease. Nature Communications. 2020;**11**(1):5886. DOI: 10.1038/s41467-020-19701-0

[67] Trompette A, Gollwitzer ES, Yadava K, Sichelstiel AK, Sprenger N, et al. Gut microbiota metabolism of dietary fiber influences allergic airway disease and hematopoiesis. Nature Medicine. 2014;**20**(2):159-166. DOI: 10.1038/nm.3444

[68] Lu H, He J, Wu Z, Xu W, Zhang H, et al. Assessment of microbiome variation during the perioperative period in liver transplant patients: A retrospective analysis. Microbial Ecology. 2013;**65**(3):781-791. DOI: 10.1007/s00248-013-0211-6

[69] Hartman AL, Lough DM, Barupal DK, Fiehn O, Fishbein T, et al. Human gut microbiome adopts an alternative state following small bowel transplantation. Proceedings of the National Academy of Sciences of the United States of America. 2009;**106**(40):17187-17192. DOI: 10.1073/pnås.0904847106

[70] Wu Q, Turturice B, Wagner S, Huang Y, Gupta PK, et al. Gut microbiota can impact chronic murine lung allograft rejection. American Journal of Respiratory Cell and Molecular Biology. 2019;**60**(1):131-134. DOI: 10.1165/rcmb.2018-0139LE

[71] Wu Q, Gupta PK, Suzuki H, Wagner SR, Zhang C, et al. CD4 T cells but not Th17 cells are required for mouse lung transplant Obliterative bronchiolitis. American Journal of Transplantation. 2015;**15**(7):1793-1804. DOI: 10.1111/ajt.13215

[72] Whiteside SA, McGinniss JE, Collman RG. The lung microbiome: Progress and promise. The Journal of Clinical Investigation. 2021;**131**(15):e150473. DOI: 10.1172/JCI150473

[73] Abbas AA, Taylor LJ, Dothard MI, Leiby JS, Fitzgerald AS, et al. Redondoviridae, a family of small, circular DNA viruses of the human Oro-respiratory tract associated with periodontitis and critical illness. Cell Host & Microbe. 2019;**25**(5):719-729.e4. DOI: 10.1016/j.chom.2019.04.001

[74] Moutsoglou DM. 2021. American Thoracic Society BEAR cage winning proposal: Microbiome transplant in pulmonary arterial hypertension. American Journal of Respiratory and Critical Care Medicine. 2022;**205**(1):13-16. DOI: 10.1164/rccm.202108-1833ED

[75] Carney SM, Clemente JC, Cox MJ, Dickson RP, Huang YJ, et al. Methods in lung microbiome research. American Journal of Respiratory Cell and

Molecular Biology. 2020;**62**(3):283-299. DOI: 10.1165/rcmb.2019-0273TR

[76] Mohgan R, Candasamy M, Mayuren J, Singh SK, Gupta G, et al. Emerging paradigms in bioengineering the lungs. Bioengineering (Basel). 2022;**9**(5):195. DOI: 10.3390/bioengineering9050195

[77] Naeem C, Mozafari M, Sefat F. Scaffolds for lung tissue engineering. In: Handbook of Tissue Engineering Scaffolds. Vol. Two. Amsterdam, The Netherlands: Elsevier; 2009. pp. 427-448

[78] De Santis MM, Bölükbas DA, Lindstedt S, Wagner DE. How to build a lung: Latest advances and emerging themes in lung bioengineering. The European Respiratory Journal. 2018;**52**(1):1601355. DOI: 10.1183/13993003.01355-2016

[79] Nikolova MP, Chavali MS. Recent advances in biomaterials for 3D scaffolds: A review. Bioactive Materials. 2019;**4**:271-292. DOI: 10.1016/j.bioactmat.2019.10.005

[80] Nichols JE, Niles JA, Cortiella J. Production and utilization of acellular lung scaffolds in tissue engineering. Journal of Cellular Biochemistry. 2012;**113**(7):2185-2192. DOI: 10.1002/jcb.24112

[81] Wanczyk H, Jensen T, Weiss DJ, Finck C. Advanced single-cell technologies to guide the development of bioengineered lungs. American Journal of Physiology. Lung Cellular and Molecular Physiology. 2021;**320**(6):L1101-L1117. DOI: 10.1152/ajplung.00089.2021

[82] Liu J, Yang BQ, Itoh A, Masood MF, Hartupee JC, et al. Impact of new UNOS allocation criteria on heart transplant practices and outcomes. Transplantation direct. 2020;**7**(1):e642. DOI: 10.1097/TXD.0000000000001088

[83] Hanff TC, Harhay MO, Kimmel SE, Molina M, Mazurek JA, et al. Trends in mechanical support use as a bridge to adult heart transplant under new allocation rules. JAMA Cardiology. 2020;**5**(6):728-729. DOI: 10.1001/jamacardio.2020.0667

[84] Zaky M, Nordan T, Kapur NK, Vest AR, DeNofrio D, et al. Impella 5.5 support beyond 50 days as bridge to heart transplant in end-stage heart failure patients. ASAIO Journal. 2022. DOI: 10.1097/MAT.0000000000001796

[85] Pahwa S, Dunbar-Matos C, Slaughter MS, Trivedi JR. Use of Impella in patients listed for heart transplantation. ASAIO Journal. 2022;**68**(6):786-790. DOI: 10.1097/MAT.0000000000001679

[86] Glazier JJ, Kaki A. The Impella device: Historical background, clinical applications and future directions. International Journal of Angiology. 2019;**28**(2):118-123. DOI: 10.1055/s-0038-1676369

[87] Monteagudo-Vela M, Panoulas V, García-Saez D, de Robertis F, Stock U, et al. Outcomes of heart transplantation in patients bridged with Impella 5.0: Comparison with native chest transplanted patients without preoperative mechanical circulatory support. Artificial Organs. 2021;**45**(3):254-262. DOI: 10.1111/aor.13816

[88] Ramzy D, Soltesz E, Anderson M. New surgical circulatory support system outcomes. ASAIO Journal. 2020;**66**(7):746-752. DOI: 10.1097/MAT.0000000000001194

[89] D'Alessandro D, Philpott J, Boeve T, Pham S, Zuckermann A. First report of the GUARDIAN registry: An international consortium examining the effect of controlled hypothermic preservation in heart transplantation.

The Journal of Heart and Lung Transplantation. 2021;**40**(4):S127

[90] Connellan M, Dhital K. Donor heart procurement from the donation after circulatory death pathway. Operative Techniques in Thoracic and Cardiovascular Surgery. 2017;**22**(1):58-67

[91] Alomari M, Garg P, Yazji JH, Wadiwala IJ, Alamouti-Fard E, et al. Is the organ care system (OCS) still the first choice with emerging new strategies for donation after circulatory death (DCD) in heart transplant? Cureus. 2022;**14**(6):e26281. DOI: 10.7759/cureus.26281

[92] Alamouti-Fard E, Garg P, Wadiwala IJ, Yazji JH, Alomari M, Hussain MWA, et al. Normothermic regional perfusion is an emerging cost-effective alternative in donation after circulatory death (DCD) in heart transplantation. Cureus. 2022;**14**(6):e26437. DOI: 10.7759/cureus.26437

[93] Benck L, Sato T, Kobashigawa J. Molecular diagnosis of rejection in heart transplantation. Circulation Journal. 2022;**86**(7):1061-1067. DOI: 10.1253/circj.CJ-21-0591

[94] Halloran PF, Reeve JP, Pereira AB, Hidalgo LG, Famulski KS. Antibody-mediated rejection, T cell-mediated rejection, and the injury-repair response: New insights from the Genome Canada studies of kidney transplant biopsies. Kidney International. 2014;**85**(2):258-264. DOI: 10.1038/ki.2013.300

[95] Halloran PF, Potena L, Van Huyen JD, Bruneval P, Leone O, et al. Building a tissue-based molecular diagnostic system in heart transplant rejection: The heart molecular microscope diagnostic (MMDx) system. The Journal of Heart and Lung Transplantation. 2017;**36**(11):1192-1200. DOI: 10.1016/j.healun.2017.05.029

[96] Parkes MD, Aliabadi AZ, Cadeiras M, Crespo-Leiro MG, Deng M, et al. An integrated molecular diagnostic report for heart transplant biopsies using an ensemble of diagnostic algorithms. The Journal of Heart and Lung Transplantation. 2019;**38**(6):636-646. DOI: 10.1016/j.healun.2019.01.1318

[97] Deng MC, Eisen HJ, Mehra MR, Billingham M, Marboe CC, et al; CARGO Investigators. Noninvasive discrimination of rejection in cardiac allograft recipients using gene expression profiling. American Journal of Transplantation. 2006;**6**(1):150-160. DOI: 10.1111/j.1600-6143.2005.01175.x

[98] Fang KC. Clinical utilities of peripheral blood gene expression profiling in the management of cardiac transplant patients. Journal of Immunotoxicology. 2007;**4**(3):209-217. DOI: 10.1080/15476910701385570

[99] Pham MX, Teuteberg JJ, Kfoury AG, Starling RC, Deng MC, et al. Gene-expression profiling for rejection surveillance after cardiac transplantation. The New England Journal of Medicine. 2010;**362**(20):1890-1900. DOI: 10.1056/NEJMoa0912965

[100] Kobashigawa J, Patel J, Azarbal B, Kittleson M, Chang D, et al. Randomized pilot trial of gene expression profiling versus heart biopsy in the first year after heart transplant: Early invasive monitoring attenuation through gene expression trial. Circulation. Heart Failure. 2015;**8**(3):557-564. DOI: 10.1161/CIRCHEARTFAILURE.114.001658

[101] Crespo-Leiro MG, Stypmann J, Schulz U, Zuckermann A, Mohacsi P, et al. Clinical usefulness of gene-expression profile to rule out acute rejection after heart transplantation: CARGO II. European Heart Journal. 2016;**37**(33):2591-2601. DOI: 10.1093/eurheartj/ehv682

[102] Amadio JM, Rodenas-Alesina E, Superina S, Kozuszko S, et al. Sparing the prod: Providing an alternative to endomyocardial biopsies with noninvasive surveillance after heart transplantation during COVID-19. CJC Open. 2022;**4**(5):479-487. DOI: 10.1016/j.cjco.2022.02.002

Chapter 8

Machine Perfusion Strategies in Liver and Renal Transplantation

Stella Vasileiadou, Nikolaos Antoniadis, Athanasios Kofinas, Konstantina-Eleni Karakasi, Georgios Katsanos and Georgios Tsoulfas

Abstract

Transplantation is the only treatment for patients with end-stage renal and hepatic disease but unfortunately, it is limited worldwide due to the organ shortage. The need to expand the donor pool with the use of donors after cardiac death (DCD) and extended criteria donors (ECD) has led to major improvements in organ preservation. From cold static storage and preservation solutions to different types of machine perfusion, the possibility of successfully transplanting a marginal organ becomes reality. In this chapter, we examine the machine perfusion methods and the advantages of new technology in minimizing ischemic injury and improving the transplant outcome. The establishment of protocols with the use of biomarkers in order to assess the transplant suitability of the graft will eventually provide the ideal opportunity to intervene and improve the quality of the organ.

Keywords: machine perfusion, liver transplantation, kidney transplantation, organ preservation, hypothermic machine perfusion, normothermic machine perfusion

1. Introduction

In this chapter, after a brief introductory reference to the definition and history of machine perfusion in transplantation, their contemporary necessity is discussed. For this purpose, two important topics such as ischemia–reperfusion injury and marginal grafts are analyzed. Subsequently, the machine perfusion strategies in liver and kidney transplantation are mentioned separately.

The review of the literature was conducted using the combination of various keywords (liver transplantation, kidney/renal transplantation, machine perfusion, hypothermic/normothermic/subnormothermic machine perfusion, ischemia–reperfusion injury, marginal grafts, extended criteria donors, donors after cardiac death, cold static storage, and organ preservation) in PubMed research database. The inclusion criteria of the articles were the English language and their relevance to the topic, which was judged by the authors after studying the abstracts.

Transplantation is the only treatment for patients with end-stage renal and hepatic disease. Despite the recent U.S. milestone of 1 million transplants until 2022, the number of patients on waiting lists remains high [1]. The great need for increment of the donor pool leads to the utilization of allografts from extended criteria donors (ECD) and donors after circulatory death (DCD). The vulnerability of these marginal grafts in ischemia–reperfusion injury (IRI) [2] revealed all the weak points of standard preservation methods and resulted in poor transplant outcomes. Moreover, the ECD and DCD kidney grafts have increased immunogenicity and as a result higher rates of rejection [3].

The combination of nonideal donors with limitations in graft evaluation results in discarded organs that further exacerbate the transplantation gap. In an attempt to find solutions, the interest of scientific community turned to preservation strategies, particularly the application of machine perfusion methods to these organs, in order to assess and make them suitable for transplantation [4, 5].

The concept of machine perfusion (MP) in the field of transplantation is not new. In 1885, the initial idea of extracorporeal circulation with the construction of a closed circulatory system [6] and 52 years later the transition from blood to chemical perfusion solutions, in order to keep organs "alive" [7], laid the foundations for the development of organ preservation. Machine perfusion in a human kidney was performed for the first time in 1967 by Belzer. The first liver transplantation in humans was performed by Starzl, with the application of a hypothermic low-flow perfusion method that used diluted blood [8, 9]. Thus, although the original concept involved room temperature and dynamic perfusion, in 1969 Collins GM changed completely the perspective, with the 12-hour preservation of canine kidneys in an iced solution, which later evolved into Collins solution with a longer preservation time [10]. Nowadays, preserving the organ in an ice box at 0–4°C, after flushing it with a cold preservation solution (usually the University of Wisconsin or Histidine-Tryptophan-Ketoglutarate solution), is the most common method worldwide. Static cold storage (SCS) has been established as the gold standard due to its simplicity, efficacy, and low cost [11]. The idea of machine perfusion was abandoned but, in the beginning of this century, gained interest again in clinical practice.

Machine perfusion is an *ex-vivo* platform where organs are connected to a pump and perfused with the solution in a controlled flow, constantly, until implantation. The main purpose is to provide essential substances and remove waste products in order to maintain cellular metabolism in a predetermined way. There is variation in machine perfusion methods in terms of temperature, oxygen and nutrient supply, preservation solutions, delivery method, duration, and time-point of perfusion. Depending on the temperature, there are three types of machine perfusion: normothermic (35.5–37.5°C), hypothermic (1–8°C), and subnormothermic (20–35.5°C) temperature with the latter sought in fewer studies [12]. Also, the variation of temperatures differs slightly in the literature.

Hypothermia reduces cellular metabolism while at the same time, the preservation solution enhances ATP production [13]. Also, the addition of oxygen restores mitochondrial oxidative activity by electron transport [14]. Hypothermic machine perfusion (HMP) has the significant advantage of safety, as in case of machine failure, the graft can easily be preserved in SCS.

The aim of reducing cold ischemia time (CIT), which is an independent risk factor for delayed graft function (DGF), has led to the development of normothermic machine perfusion (NMP). During this method, the reperfusion phase after ischemia time takes place in an artificial environment as close as possible to physiological conditions (temperature and oxygen), in order to avoid the inflammatory process and the destructive injury, it causes to the graft. Normothermia has the important advantage of assessing the graft in real-time, as bile and urine are produced by liver and kidney grafts, respectively [15]. On the other hand, it is a more complicated and costly procedure as it requires a sufficient amount of oxygen, oxygen carriers, and necessary substances for the graft function [16]. In an effort to limit the use of human blood products with red blood cells or plasma, the development of extracellular oxygen carriers began [17].

Subnormothermic machine perfusion (SNMP) is an intermediate state between hypothermic and normothermic conditions, maintaining low cellular energy demands and mitochondrial activity, while the organ is still "alive." This method is simpler than NMP as red blood cells are not necessary [18]. Although SNMP started as a promising technique, disappointing results in a porcine kidney model prevented its further clinical application. The SNMP group had increased rates of renal and tubular injury than the NMP group [19]. Currently, it is still at an experimental stage in both liver and kidney transplantation with important clinical prospects.

Controlled oxygenated rewarming (COR) is an alternative perfusion method that focuses on transitioning the graft from hypothermia to normothermia by gradually increasing the temperature (from 8–20°C). Mitochondrial function can be affected by rapid temperature change when the graft is reperfused after cold ischemic preservation. In particular, the opening of the mitochondrial permeability transition pore contributes in a destructive way to the occurrence of IRI. COR allows smooth recovery of mitochondrial function and studies have shown its feasibility in clinical application in liver and kidney transplantation [20, 21].

In the last decade, many studies have been published on different models of machine perfusion and large clinical trials in humans have been performed, changing the concept of preservation in transplantation. From procurement to transplantation, the reasons for this development, in addition to the increasing use of ECD or DCD grafts, are the comprehension of the complicated biological pathways and phenomena such as IRI.

1.1 Ischemia: Reperfusion injury

During organ procurement, the blood supply to the organs is interrupted, and after implantation or *ex-situ* normothermic machine perfusion of the grafts, it is restored. This process, defined as ischemia–reperfusion injury, leads to cell death in an oxidative environment and production of reactive oxygen species (ROS) [2].

IRI consists of three phases and each of them causes a different effect on the organ. First, it is the ischemic phase, when the blood and oxygen supply of the organ is inhibited. Dramatic depletion of ATP unregulates sodium-potassium ATPases in cell membranes, resulting in increased calcium concentration and acidic pH [22, 23]. It is of notice that the type of donor (donation after brain death or after circulatory death) plays an important role in ischemia injury to the graft [24]. Second, it is the reperfusion phase, when ischemic tissues are reoxygenated and as a result release ROS, that is mainly formed in complex 1 - mitochondrial respiratory chain [25]. Furthermore, in liver grafts, disorders in the mitochondrial permeability transition pore (MPTP) allow the release of danger-associated molecular patterns (DAMPs) from the nucleus [26], which interact with Toll-like receptors (TLRs) and activate Kupffer cells [27]. Finally, a prolonged period of inflammation is established where important liver microstructures are deranged. For example, damage to the endothelial glycocalyx or the combination of increased vasoconstrictive agents and decreased nitric oxide levels deteriorates the microcirculation and raises the risk of early allograft dysfunction (EAD) [28, 29]. Third is the late injury phase, which follows the release of ROS and continues the cascade of cytotoxic events with the activation of resident and recruited immune cells [30].

IRI is globally independent risk factor in transplantation and is related to acute rejection, postreperfusion syndrome, DGF, and primary non-function (PNF) [31]. The standard static cold storage was an inferior preservation method for kidneys [32] and failed to protect marginal livers from the effects of ischemia–reperfusion injury [33], so the need for a different strategy was imperative. Continuous machine perfusion circulation of metabolic substances and removal of inflammatory products, such as toxins and cytokines [34], reduce the degree of graft injury, for example, to the liver's deep peribiliary glands and stroma [35].

1.2 Marginal grafts

As already mentioned, the use of suboptimal grafts is constantly increasing due to the transplant gap between the donor pool and the recipient waiting list. Marginal liver grafts are organs with an increased chance of failure or PNF after transplantation. Also, the definition includes cases where diseases can be transmitted from the donor to the recipient [36]. Usually, high risk liver grafts come from donors with factors such as: liver macrosteatosis, cardiac death, advanced age, long stay in the intensive care unit, infections and malignancies.

Macrosteatosis is not a prohibitive factor for transplantation if the percentage is <30% but the fatty liver is considered to have worse postoperative outcomes than grafts without steatosis [37]. DCD livers due to prolonged warm ischemia time are susceptible to ischemic-type biliary lesions. Microcirculation disorders, during IRI, cause damage to the arterial plexus of the biliary tree, so there is high risk of biliary strictures after the transplantation [38]. Advanced age has negative effects on liver reserves, so injury after reperfusion is more serious and increases the risk of post-transplant complications [39].

Machine perfusion techniques appear to benefit these borderline livers most, with characteristics such as macrosteatosis >30%, DCD donors, donors >60 years old, cold ischemia time > 8-10 h, warm ischemia time > 30 min, insufficient *in situ* perfusion, prolonged organ procurement, and generally discarded grafts due to eliminated transaminases or any nonvascular problem [40, 41].

Different scoring systems have been developed to predict graft survival: Survival outcomes following liver transplantation (SOFT), donor risk index (DRI), Eurotransplant-DRI, etc. Clinical parameters (cardiac arrest >15 min, age > 55 years, BMI >30), laboratory results (AST, ALT, HBV, and HCV), ICU conditions (days, drugs, and infections) and of course histology after biopsy are included and considered in the transplant decision. Finally, nonheart beating and DCD donors are ECDs by definition [42].

The definition of borderline kidneys, which actually includes donor risk factors for kidney transplants, is derived from living donors, as in the early stages were mainly associated with risks to the recipient [43]. The Kidney donor risk index (KDRI) is a practical tool for predicting the posttransplant outcome. Factors such as weight, height, race, history of diabetes, hepatitis C status, and DCD are included [44]. The OPTN-approved criteria for ECD kidneys consider the following donor parameters: age, cerebrovascular accident as the cause of death, history of hypertension, and creatinine level [45].

Also, acute kidney injury or extracorporeal membrane oxygenation (ECMO) prior to organ retrieval significantly affects the graft quality [46, 47].

2. Machine perfusion of the liver

2.1 Hypothermic machine perfusion

During hypothermic machine perfusion, the liver graft is perfused with a preservation solution, mainly University of Wisconsin (UW) or Vasosol (modified UW), usually at 4–11°C. In this way, the graft takes essential substances and eliminates waste products [40, 48]. The pO2 level is 20 kPa, as no additional oxygen is provided. HMP clinical series was first published in 2010, as a safe and effective perfusion system by James Guarrera [49].

In hypothermic conditions, deceleration of cellular metabolism and cryoprotection, prepare the liver graft for the time of reperfusion. HMP provides protection to the graft in a complicated and not completely clarified way, as far as ischemia–reperfusion injury is concerned. Studies have shown that it has positive effects on mitochondrial complexes and increases cellular energy, leading to metabolism of molecules such as succinate [50, 51].

Also, livers perfused under hypothermic conditions had less of the ultrastructural effects seen in SCS. The number of CD68+ macrophages and, in general, inflammatory injury agents were significantly decreased, as shown by measurements at the end of preservation and after graft reperfusion [51, 52].

During hypothermic oxygenated machine perfusion (HOPE), the pO2 level is 60–100 kPa, and in this technique additional perfusate oxygen is provided to the graft. Oxygen is diluted in the perfusion fluid so there is no need for oxygen carriers [53]. Oxygenation in hypothermic conditions restores mitochondrial function and promotes metabolic activity. As a result, the reduction of ROS and succinate does not lead to further damage in mitochondrial function [54, 55].

HOPE was initially used in a clinical setting in 2014, where Maastricht Type III-DCD liver grafts were treated and subsequently assessed [56]. A matched case analysis of DCD livers compared HOPE treatment with standard SCS. 25 HOPE livers had fewer biliary complications and better 1-year graft survival than 50 SCS livers, but with longer cold ischemic time in the last group [57]. HOPE-DCD livers showed a reduced risk of acute rejection and improved 5-year graft survival in a recent study with the same comparators (94% in HOPE DCD vs. 78% in SCS DCD). They also have better laboratory results (INR and lactates on the first day) and fewer postoperative complications [58]. Moreover, HOPE treatment proved beneficial in macrosteatotic livers and has a positive impact on graft function and survival compared to the unperfused group [59]. Similarly, grafts from donors with advanced age seem to have good results with HOPE treatment. In two transplantations with octogenarian grafts, this perfusion technique promoted the recovery process after IRI and reduced hospitalization [60].

The hypothermic machine perfusion uses either the portal vein alone or the portal vein and hepatic artery together. The dual perfusion with oxygen is called dual flow hypothermic oxygenated perfusion (D-HOPE) and attempted to optimize the oxygenation of the biliary system. D-HOPE DCD livers had low peak ALT and bilirubin levels compared with SCS, but no difference in patient and 1-year graft survival. Perfusion pressure is also a technical detail of great importance during machine perfusion. High pressure leads to additional damage at endothelial cells, so the desired levels are 20–30 mmHg in the hepatic artery and 3–5 mmHg in the portal vein during HMP [61].

A meta-analysis of 12 studies comparing HMP and SCS in liver grafts showed the superiority of HMP in reducing posttransplant AST and ALT serum levels, early allograft dysfunction, total biliary complications, and ischemic cholangiopathy. No statistical significance was observed in outcomes for primary nonfunction, hepatic artery thrombosis, postreperfusion syndrome, patient survival, and liver graft survival (1 month, 6 months, and 1 year) [62]. An additional advantage of HMP is that in case of pump failure, the organ can be stored in cold static conditions, so it is a safe perfusion method.

The viability assessment during HMP is challenging because of metabolic deceleration and absence of bile production. However, there is a growing interest in the literature for potential markers during HMP and HOPE. Peak AST after transplantation was found to be associated with AST and LDH levels after 2 h of perfusion [49]. Also, cellular ATP concentration during D-HOPE appears to be related to liver posttransplant function at a biochemical level [61]. A recent study by Muller et al. discovered a new mitochondrial biomarker that can be counted by spectroscope after 30–45 min of HOPE. Flavin mitochondrial mononucleotide (FMN) is easily detected in HOPE perfusate and can predict graft function and possible complications before implantation [63].

2.2 Normothermic machine perfusion

Normothermic machine perfusion uses temperatures between 35 and 38°C and components from blood products such as erythrocytes. Oxygenators are necessary and dual perfusion (portal and arterial) is performed. The aim is to mimic the physiologic environment so that the metabolism and function of the liver graft being maintained. The first clinical introduction was in 2016 when a phase-1 clinical trial was published [64]. Minimizing clod ischemia time enables long preservation of the liver graft without injury. In fact, a recent protocol described a metabolic, active, and functional human liver after 7 days of NMP [65].

The combination of HOPE and NMP versus NMP in nontransplanted livers was studied by the Birmingham group. The HOPE/NMP livers showed lower indicators of inflammation and better recovery of their metabolic rate [66]. According to the first prospective multicenter randomized controlled trial, the use of NMP (121 livers) instead of SCS (101 livers) increases the utilization of grafts by 50%. NMP despite the longer preservation time (11.9 vs. 7.7 h) reduced the grade of graft injury as seen by the low levels of AST and EAD, in both DCD and DBD livers. However, there was no superiority of NMP in PNF, biliary complications, ischemic cholangiopathy, graft, and patient survival [67].

The great advantage of NMP is the ability to evaluate the graft during preservation time. Observation of liver parameters such as bile production with laboratory test results, such as transaminases, lactate, glucose, and pH, have created scoring systems to aid in the transplant decision. Perfusate lactate, bile production, vascular flows, and liver appearance of five rejected livers were evaluated during NMP (after SCS), and finally transplanted with good outcomes [68]. In a study in 23 human livers, biochemical parameters of bile were examined after 6 hours of NMP and compared with the grade of bile duct injury. Biliary bicarbonate, pH, glucose, and bile/perfusate glucose ratio were identified as potential biomarkers of posttransplant cholangiopathy [69].

2.3 Subnormothermic machine perfusion

Subnormothermic machine perfusion is a method that uses temperatures between HMP and NMP, usually 21–25°C, and an oxygenated preservation solution such as HOPE. This subphysiologic temperature, on one hand, reduces the metabolic rate but, on the other hand, the graft is warm enough to allow viability assessment [70].

Three hours of SNMP in seven discarded human livers showed satisfactory bile production and liver function [71] but the study did not include posttransplant outcomes in order to determine the favorable effect of SNMP.

2.4 Controlled oxygenated rewarming

In an experimental animal study, a gradual raise in temperature (up to 20°C) with simultaneous oxygenated perfusion was performed for 90 min after a period of end-ischemia HMP. Posttransplant peak transaminase level was lower, and 6 months of patient survival was higher in the COR group compared with the control group [72]. Combined protocols, such as DHOPE-COR-NMP used in discarded livers, have significantly increased the number of transplantable grafts [73].

2.5 Therapeutics in machine perfusion methods

During machine perfusion, in addition to the standard enrichment of the preservation solution (glucose, heparine, insulin, antibiotics, maybe oxygen, and nutrients), agents targeting graft recondition can be added. Machine Perfusion therapeutic agents aim to improve the marginal graft to follow a successful transplantation. The unique advantage of this *ex vivo* procedure is that the agents are washed out of the graft and cannot interact with the recipient's immune system. Defatting cocktails that increase lipolysis, vasodilators with vascular protective effects, and gene therapies with specific targets and without side effects are just several possible treatments for a marginal liver graft.

2.5.1 Defatting agents

In a porcine model, 48 h of NMP in steatotic livers resulted in higher metabolism (triglyceride, glucose, and urea in the perfusate) and less lipid detection in the tissue (histologically demonstrated) [74]. In another rodent model with steatotic grafts, 3 hours of NMP with the addition of a defatting cocktail showed a reduction of lipids in the cells with a raise in lipid mobility at the gene level [75]. The defatting cocktail was tested on discarded human grafts with good outcomes compared to the control group. Triglycerides accumulation and the grade of macrovesicular steatosis were significantly reduced [76].

2.5.2 Vasodilators

Prostaglandin E1 is a vasodilator with fibrin clot dissolution activity, which has been shown to meliorate microcirculation injury. Rodent studies where PGE1 is used in NMP verified the beneficial effect on treated livers. The levels of aspartate and alanine aminotransferase were decreased and the bile production was higher [77, 78]. Nitroglycerin and prostaglandin E1 were contained in the Vasosol solution used in the first clinical trial of HMP in human livers [79]. Apart from PGE1, prostacyclin had the same advantages in treated porcine livers [80]. Another porcine transplant study researched the effect of BQ123 and verapamil as vasodilators and noticed that treated livers had better flow in the hepatic artery [81].

2.5.3 Gene modulation agents

Antisense oligonucleotides (ASOs) and siRNA are auspicious gene agents that can have specific targets without the need for viral convection. Silencing of miRNA-122 by ASO resulted in reduced HCV activity in a porcine study [82]. Despite the fact that antiviral medication is widespread and efficient, this finding is important in the evolution of MP therapeutics. siRNAs can have multiple targets such as Fas pathway, p53, RelB, TNF-a, and proapoptotic caspases. All these targets are associated with different aspects of IRI and can potentially protect livers, as shown in animal models under normothermic or hypothermic conditions [83–85].

2.5.4 Others

Anti-inflammatory agents (alprostadil, n- acetylcysteine, carbon monoxide, and sevoflurane) used under subnormothermic or hypothermic conditions, especially the NLRP3 inflammasome inhibitor mcc950 [86], enkephalin, which is a Δ-opioid agonist treated rat livers under NMP [87], and human liver stem cells in an extracellular form [88], significantly reduced IRI markers.

3. Machine perfusion of the kidney

3.1 Hypothermic machine perfusion

HMP has been established as a safe and effective preservation method with benefits in kidney transplantation. In one of the first RCTs with 336 deceased donors, nonoxygenated HMP was superior to CSC in reducing DGF and increasing 1-year graft survival, regardless of donor type [32]. This publication integrated HMP into daily clinical practice. Afterward, the good short-term results (DGF and 1-month kidney function) of HMP were also confirmed in DCD kidneys. Regarding long-term outcomes, the 164 kidney transplants (82 HMP vs. 82 SCS) had no significant difference in 1-year graft survival [89].

The addition of oxygen and the development of HOPE showed promising results. Application of HOPE in a rodent study significantly decreased markers of reperfusion injury (IL-6, ENO, and TNF-alpha) after kidney transplantation [90]. In a recent meta-analysis, PNF and DGF were significantly reduced in HMP kidneys compared with SCS, but no difference in acute rejection was observed. Also, one-year graft survival was longer in the HMP group [91].

Although the benefit of HMP over SCS has been proven, a large randomized clinical trial COPE-POMP, which evaluated ECD kidneys stored on ice and then perfused in oxygenated hypothermic conditions for 2 hours before implantation, showed no advantages in graft survival (3 months and 1 year) and function (PNF and DGF). These results may be associated with the use of HMP in different centers [92]. Another recent RCT, COPE-COMPARE, compared oxygenated HMP with nonoxygenated HMP in Maastricht III DCD kidneys (50 years and older). The first group improved renal function while decreasing posttransplant complications and acute rejections [93].

The ideal duration and timepoint of HMP are under research, with most studies using end-ischemia time. This phase is practical as the graft is transported on ice and assessed prior to transplantation. In a clinical study of 66 ECD kidneys subjected to end-ischemic perfusion for 369 minutes, the percentage of DGF was 0 versus 9.3% in the contralateral kidneys preserved in SCS [94].

Several potential biomarkers for graft assessment have been studied. The levels of glutathione S-transferase (GST), N-acetyl-beta-D- glucosaminidase (NAG), heart-type fatty acid-binding protein (H-FABP), or LDH measured in the perfusate during MP and are related to DGF [95–97]. Parameters in HMP, such as resistance and flow, are used in scoring systems to assess kidney quality and risk of DGF [98]. It is noteworthy that CIT, as an independent risk factor in graft function after transplantation, increases the percentage of DGF as hours of cold ischemia pass. As the study of the data from the "Machine Perfusion Trial" showed, if CIT was above 10 hours, DGF was not reduced by HMP [99].

3.2 Normothermic machine perfusion

The first clinical application of NMP (35 min after 11 hours of SCS) in human kidney transplantation was in 2011 with good postoperative results [100]. A larger clinical study compared 18 ECD kidneys that underwent NMP (for approximately 63 min) with matched ECD kidneys that were preserved on ice. DGF was lower in the NMP group (5.6 vs. 36.2%) but 1-year graft survival was comparable in both groups [101].

The advantages of preserving a kidney in normothermic conditions are many. Cold ischemic injury is minimized as aerobic metabolism and renal functions are restarted [102]. The preservation time is investigated in the literature. In a recent study, discarded human kidneys underwent 24 h of NMP using urine recirculation with stable or slightly better tubular function after histopathological assessment [103].

The observation of the graft is feasible and provides the opportunity for assessment.

Parameters, such as total urine output, renal blood flow, and macroscopic perfusion during NMP, are used in score systems to evaluate the graft quality and "transplantability" [104]. Of course, therapies and agents that improve the condition of the graft prior to transplantation are feasible in normothermic preservation. A functional organ in NMP is more easily modified than in hypothermic conditions where cellular mechanisms are under-functioning.

3.3 Therapeutics in machine perfusion

3.3.1 Hypothermic conditions

Mesenchymal stem cells (MSC) and their extracellular vesicles, which have been used in a rat model where the kidneys underwent HMP, have a potential protective role in the perfusion process. The results showed increased activation of enzymes related to cell metabolism and membrane permeability [105]. Carbon monoxide-releasing molecule 401 (CORM-401) decreased IRI markers and improved graft function [106]. Anticoagulative agents, such as thrombalexin and heparin conjugate, have been tested to improve microcirculation, with positive outcomes in the kidneys [107, 108].

3.3.2 Normothermic conditions

Application of MSCs to NMP had a suppressive role in the inflammatory process, in human kidneys [109]. Erythropoietin and its derivative, cyclic helix B peptide (CHBP), can reduce inflammatory agents, such as caspase-3 and IL-1β, providing renoprotection against IRI and improving urine production of the kidney. Recently, a mouse kidney model defined the role of endoplasmic reticulum stress (ERS) in IRI and pointed out the therapeutic potential of CHBP with CHOP (an indicator of ERS) as a biomarker

[110–112]. Also, nanoparticles can be used as drug-delivered agents in blocking or preventing events of inflammation at a molecular level. For example, a possible target is the vascular cells of the graft's endothelium that are mainly damaged by IRI and performed antidonor antibodies. Nanoparticles, with the presence of anti-CD 31 antibodies, can target endothelial cells and deliver therapeutic agents during NMP [113].

4. Conclusion

Banking organs on a worldwide scale after quality tests would be the ideal method of organ preservation in order to select the perfect-match recipient and then proceed to scheduled surgery [114]. This goal has been achieved in stem cell transplantation and important achievements are taking place in solid organ transplantation, through the development of organ preservation with machine perfusion. Starting with animal experiments and, subsequently, with human clinical studies and randomized controlled trials, machine perfusion is an alternative that still has a lot to offer in solid organ transplantation.

The advantages of MP in short-term outcomes of transplantation are dependent on the preservation method but also the beneficial effects in long-term organ function are continuously demonstrated. It is a platform where, beyond quality, the immunogenicity of the graft could be studied and modified according to the profile of the recipient [103]. The specific targets and the lower dosages, which can be achieved using MP therapeutics agents compared to conventional systemic pharmacological agents, open a new chapter in marginal graft utilization. This may in the future help change the transplant process to a more personalized medicine approach.

New MP technology reveals new perspectives in transplant logistics. Graft evaluation leads to more transplantable organs perhaps in more complex recipients. The prolonged time of preservation provides the opportunity for preoperative planning and elective surgery in day time.

"*Which perfusion technique enables the highest utilization rate of otherwise discarded livers with the best available outcomes, regarding complications, graft- and patient survival*" [115]. This question, which could concern the kidney as well, remains to be answered. So far, there is no evidence of the superiority of a preservation strategy. Randomized clinical trials with combined perfusion protocols may provide the answer to the ideal approach in solid organ transplantation.

Author details

Stella Vasileiadou*, Nikolaos Antoniadis, Athanasios Kofinas,
Konstantina-Eleni Karakasi, Georgios Katsanos and Georgios Tsoulfas
Organ Transplant Unit, Hippokration General Hospital, Aristotle University of Thessaloniki, Thessaloniki, Greece

*Address all correspondence to: stvasileiadou@gmail.com

References

[1] Available from: https://unos.org

[2] Chouchani ET, Pell VR, Gaude E, Aksentijević D, Sundier SY, Robb EL, et al. Ischaemic accumulation of succinate controls reperfusion injury through mitochondrial ROS. Nature. 2014;**515**:431-435

[3] Rao PS, Ojo A. The alphabet soup of kidney transplantation: SCD, DCD, ECD–fundamentals for the practicing nephrologist. Clinical Journal of the American Society of Nephrology. 2009;**4**:1827-1831. DOI: 10.2215/CJN.02270409

[4] Meister FA, Czigany Z, Bednarsch J, Bocker J, Amygdalos I, Morales Santana DA, et al. Hypothermic oxygenated machine perfusion of extended criteria kidney allografts from brain dead donors: Protocol for a prospective pilot study. JMIR Research Protocols. 2019;**8**:e14622

[5] Czigany Z, Schoning W, Ulmer TF, Bednarsch J, Amygdalos I, Cramer T, et al. Hypothermic oxygenated machine perfusion (HOPE) for orthotopic liver transplantation of human liver allografts from extended criteria donors (ECD) in donation after brain death (DBD): A prospective multicentre randomised controlled trial (HOPE ECD-DBD). BMJ Open. 2017;**7**:e017558

[6] Okiljević B, ŠuŠak S, Redžek A, Rosić M, Velicki L. Development of cardiopulmonary bypass–a historical review. Srpski Arhiv za Celokupno Lekarstvo. 2016;**144**:670-675

[7] Carrel A. The culture of whole organs: I. technique of the culture of the thyroid gland. The Journal of Experimental Medicine. 1937;**65**:515-526

[8] Brettschneider L, Daloze PM, Huguet C, et al. Successful orthotopic transplantation of liver homografts after eight to twenty-five hours preservation. Surgical Forum. 1967;**18**:376-378

[9] Starzl TE, Groth CG, Brettschneider L, et al. Extended survival in 3 cases of orthotopic homotransplantation of the human liver. Surgery. 1968;**63**:549-563

[10] Jing L, Yao L, Zhao M, Peng LP, Liu M. Organ preservation: From the past to the future. Acta Pharmacologica Sinica. 2018;**39**:845-857. DOI: 10.1038/aps.2017.182

[11] Liu WP, Humphries AL, Russell R, Stoddard LD, Moretz WH, Moretz WH. 48-hour storage of canine kidneys after brief perfusion with Collins' solution. Annals of Surgery. 1971;**173**:748-757

[12] Rojas-Pena A, Bartlett RH. Ex situ organ preservation: The temperature paradigm. Transplantation. 2018;**102**:554-556. DOI: 10.1097/TP.0000000000002081

[13] Karangwa SA, Dutkowski P, Fontes P, Friend PJ, Guarrera JV, Markmann JF, et al. Machine perfusion of donor livers for transplantation: A proposal for standard- ized nomenclature and reporting guide- lines. American Journal of Transplantation. 2016;**16**(10):2932-2942

[14] Stegemann J, Minor T. Energy charge restoration, mitochondrial protection and reversal of preservation induced liver injury by hypothermic oxygenation prior to reperfusion. Cryobiology. 2009;**58**(3):331-336

[15] Minor T, von Horn C, Paul A. Role of tem- perature in reconditioning and evaluation of cold preserved kidney and

liver grafts. Current Opinion in Organ Transplantation. 2017;**22**(3):267-267

[16] Hessheimer AJ, Fondevila C. Liver perfusion devices: How close are we to widespread application? Current Opinion in Organ Transplantation. 2017;**22**(2):105-111

[17] Fontes P, Lopez R, van der Plaats A, Vodovotz Y, Minervini M, Scott V, et al. Liver preservation with machine perfusion and a newly developed cell-free oxygen carrier solution under subnormothermic conditions. American Journal of Transplantation. 2015;**15**(2):381-394

[18] Selten J, Schlegel A, de Jonge J, Dutkowski P. Hypo- and normothermic perfusion of the liver: Which way to go? Best Practice & Research. Clinical Gastroenterology. 2017;**31**(2):171-179

[19] Adams TD, Patel M, Hosgood SA, Nicholson ML. Lowering perfusate temperature from 37 to 32°C diminishes function in a porcine model of ex vivo kidney perfusion. Transplantation direct. 2017;**3**:e140

[20] Schopp I, Reissberg E, Lüer B, Efferz P, Minor T. Controlled rewarming after hypothermia: Adding a new principle to renal preservation. Clinical and Translational Science. 2015;**8**:475-478

[21] Hoyer DP, Mathé Z, Gallinat A, Canbay AC, Treckmann JW, Rauen U, et al. Controlled oxygenated rewarming of cold stored livers prior to transplantation. Transplantation. 2016;**100**:147-152

[22] Carini R, Bellomo G, Benedetti A, Fulceri R, Gamberucci A, Parola M, et al. Alteration of Na+ homeostasis as a critical step in the development of irreversible hepatocyte injury after adenosine triphosphate depletion. Hepatology. 1995;**21**:1089-1098

[23] Zaouali MA, Ben Abdennebi H, Padrissa-Altes S, Mahfoudh-Boussaid A, Rosello-Catafau J. Pharmacological strategies against cold ischemia reperfusion injury. Expert Opinion on Pharmacotherapy. 2010;**11**:537-555

[24] Hessheimer AJ, Garcia-Valdecasas JC, Fondevila C. Abdominal regional in-situ perfusion in donation after circulatory determination of death donors. Current Opinion in Organ Transplantation. 2016;**21**:322-328

[25] Niatsetskaya ZV, Sosunov SA, Matsiukevich D, Utkina-Sosunova IV, Ratner VI, Starkov AA, et al. The oxygen free radicals originating from mitochondrial complex I contribute to oxidative brain injury following hypoxia-ischemia in neonatal mice. The Journal of Neuroscience. 2012;**32**:3235-3244

[26] Hoyer DP, Mathe Z, Gallinat A, Canbay AC, Treckmann JW, Rauen U, et al. Controlled oxygenated rewarming of cold stored livers prior to transplantation: First clinical application of a new concept. Transplantation. 2016;**100**:147-152

[27] van Golen RF, Reiniers MJ, Olthof PB, van Gulik TM, Heger M. Sterile inflammation in hepatic ischemia/reperfusion injury: Present concepts and potential therapeutics. Journal of Gastroenterology and Hepatology. 2013;**28**:394-400

[28] Koo A, Komatsu H, Tao G, Inoue M, Guth PH, Kaplowitz N. Contribution of no-reflow phenomenon to hepatic injury after ischemia-reperfusion: Evidence for a role for superoxide anion. Hepatology. 1992;**15**:507-514

[29] Schiefer J, Peter F, Stefan K, Bianca T, Dagmar K, Lorenz K, et al.

Glycocalyx damage within human liver grafts correlates with graft injury and postoperative graft function after Orthotopic liver transplantation. Transplantation. 2020;**104**(1):72-78. DOI: 10.1097/TP.0000000000002838

[30] Stewart RK, Dangi A, Huang C, Murase N, Kimura S, Stolz DB, et al. A novel mouse model of depletion of stellate cells clarifies their role in ischemia/reperfusion- and endotoxin-induced acute liver injury. Journal of Hepatology. 2014;**60**:298-305

[31] Land WG. The role of postischemic reperfusion injury and other nonantigen-dependent inflammatory pathways in transplantation. Transplantation. 2005;**79**:505-514

[32] Moers C, Smits JM, Maathuis M-HJ, et al. Machine perfusion or cold storage in deceased-donor kidney transplantation. The New England Journal of Medicine. 2009;**360**:7

[33] Quillin RC 3rd, Guarrera JV. Hypothermic machine perfusion in liver transplantation. Liver Transplantation. 2018;**24**:276-281. DOI: 10.1002/lt.25004

[34] Marecki H, Bozorgzadeh A, Porte RJ, Leuvenink HG, Uygun K, Martins NP. Liver ex situ machine perfusion preservation: A review of the methodology and results of large animal studies and clinical trials. Liver Transplantation. 2017;**23**:679-695. DOI: 10.1002/lt.24751

[35] van Rijn R, van Leeuwen OB, Matton APM, Burlage LC, Wiersema-Buist JMC, van den Heuvel RHJ, et al. Porte: Hypothermic oxygenated machine perfusion reduces bile duct reperfusion injury after transplantation of donation after circulatory death livers. Liver Transplantation. 2018;24:655-664. DOI: 10.1002/lt.25023

[36] Attia M, Silva MA, Mirza DF. The marginal liver donor—An update. Transplant International. 2008;**21**:713-724

[37] European association for the study of the liver. EASL clinical practice guidelines: Liver transplantation. Journal of Hepatology. 2016;**64**(2):433-485

[38] Jay CL, Lyuksemburg V, Ladner DP, Wang E, Caicedo JC, Holl JL, et al. Ischemic cholangiopathy after controlled donation after cardiac death liver transplantation: A meta-analysis. Annals of Surgery. 2011;**253**:259-264

[39] Detelich D, Markmann JF. The dawn of liver perfusion machines. Current Opinion in Organ Transplantation. 2018;**23**:151-161

[40] Czigany Z, Lurje I, Tolba RH, et al. Machine perfusion for liver transplantation in the era of marginal organs-new kids on the block. Liver International. 2019;**39**:228-249

[41] Czigany Z, Tacke F, Lurje G. Evolving trends in machine liver perfusion: Comments on clinical end points and selection criteria. Gastroenterology. 2019;**157**:1166-1167

[42] Jimenez-Romero C, Caso Maestro O, Cambra Molero F, Justo Alonso I, Alegre Torrado C, Manrique Municio A, et al. Using old liver grafts for liver transplantation: Where are the limits? World Journal of Gastroenterology. 2014;**20**:10691-10702. DOI: 10.3748/wjg.v20.i31.10691

[43] Reese PP, Caplan AL, Kesselheim AS, Bloom RD. Creating a medical, ethical, and legal framework for complex living kidney donors. Clinical Journal of the American Society of Nephrology. 2006;**1**:1148-1153. DOI: 10.2215/CJN.02180606

[44] Schamberger B, Lohmann D, Sollinger D, Stein R, Lutz J. Association of kidney donor risk index with the outcome after kidney transplantation in the eurotransplant senior program. Annals of Transplantation. 2018;**23**:775-781. DOI: 10.12659/AOT.909622

[45] Metzger RA, Delmonico FL, Feng S, Port FK, Wynn JJ, Merion RM. Expanded criteria donors for kidney transplantation. American Journal of Transplantation. 2003;**3**(Suppl. 4):114-125. DOI: 10.1034/j.1600-6143.3.s4.11.x

[46] Domagala P, Gorski L, Wszola M, Kieszek R, Diuwe P, Goralski P, et al. Successful transplantation of kidneys from deceased donors with terminal acute kidney injury. Renal Failure. 2019;**41**:167-174. DOI: 10.1080/0886022X.2019.1590209

[47] Bronchard R, Durand L, Legeai C, Cohen J, Guerrini P, Bastien O. Brain-dead donors on extracorporeal membrane oxygenation. Critical Care Medicine. 2017;**45**:1734-1741. DOI: 10.1097/CCM.0000000000002564

[48] Schlegel A, Kron P, Dutkowski P. Hypothermicoxygenatedliverperfusion: Basic mechanisms and clinical application. Current Transplantation Reports. 2015;**2**:52-62

[49] Guarrera JV, Henry SD, Samstein B, Reznik E, Musat C, Lukose TI, et al. Hypothermic machine preservation facilitates successful transplantation of "orphan" extended criteria donor livers. American Journal of Transplantation. 2015;**15**:161-169

[50] Nachber E, Tulipan J, Stone J, Bae C, Reznik L, Kato T, et al. Hypothermic machine preservation reduces molecular markers of ischemia/reperfusion injury in human liver transplantation. American Journal of Transplantation. 2012;**12**:2477-2486

[51] Schlegel A, de Rougemont O, Graf R, Clavien PA, Dutkowski P. Protective mechanisms of end-ischemic cold machine perfusion in DCD liver grafts. Journal of Hepatology. 2013;**58**:278-286

[52] Henry SD, Nachber E, Tulipan J, Stone J, Bae C, Reznik L, et al. Hypothermic machine preservation reduces molecular markers of ischemia/reperfusion injury in human liver transplantation. American Journal of Transplantation. 2012;**12**:2477-2486

[53] de Rougemont O, Breitenstein S, Leskosek B, Weber A, Graf R, Clavien PA, et al. One hour hypothermic oxygenated perfusion (HOPE) protects nonviable liver allografts donated after cardiac death. Annals of Surgery. 2009;**250**:674-683

[54] Yoshikawa R, Matsuno N, Morito N, et al. Evaluation using an isolated reperfusion model for porcine liver donated after cardiac death preserved with oxygenated hypothermic machine perfusion. Annals of Transplantation. 2018;**23**:822-827

[55] Kron P, Schlegel A, Mancina L, Clavien PA, Dutkowski P. Hypothermic oxygenated perfusion (HOPE) for fatty liver grafts in rats and humans. Journal of Hepatology. 2018;**68**(1):82-91

[56] Dutkowski P, Schlegel A, de Oliveira M, Mullhaupt B, Neff F, Clavien PA. HOPE for human liver grafts obtained from donors after cardiac death. Journal of Hepatology. 2014;**60**:765-772

[57] Dutkowski P, Polak WG, Muiesan P, et al. First comparison of hypo- thermic oxygenated perfusion versus static cold storage of human donation after cardiac death liver transplants: An international-matched case analysis. Annals of Surgery. 2015;**262**:764-770

[58] Schlegel A, Muller X, Kalisvaart M, et al. Outcomes of DCD liver transplantation using organs treated by hypothermic oxygenated perfusion before implantation. Journal of Hepatology. 2019;**70**(1):50-57

[59] Kron P, Schlegel A, Mancina L, Clavien PA, Dutkowski P. Hypothermic oxygenated perfusion (HOPE) for fatty liver grafts in rats and humans. Journal of Hepatology. 21 Sep 2017:**S0168-8278**(17):32268-7

[60] Rayar M, Maillot B, Bergeat D, et al. A preliminary clinical experience using hypo- thermic oxygenated machine perfusion for rapid recovery of octogenarian liver grafts. Progress in Transplantation. 2018;**29**(1):97-98. DOI: 10.1177/1526924818817072

[61] van Rijn R, Karimian N, Matton APM, Burlage LC, Westerkamp AC, van den Berg AP, et al. Dual hypothermic oxygenated machine perfusion in liver transplants donated after circulatory death. The British Journal of Surgery. 2017;**104**:907-917. DOI: 10.1002/bjs.10515

[62] Jia J, Nie Y, Li J, Xie H, Zhou L, Yu J, et al. Systematic Review and Meta-Analysis of Machine Perfusion vs Static Cold Storage of Liver Allografts on Liver Transplantation Outcomes: The Future Direction of Graft Preservation. Front Med (Lausanne). 12 May 2020;**7**:135

[63] Muller X, Schlegel A, Kron P, Eshmuminov D, Wurdinger M, Meierhofer D, et al. Novel real-time prediction of liver graft function during hypothermic oxygenated machine perfusion before liver transplantation. Annals of Surgery. 2019;**270**:783-790

[64] Ravikumar R, Jassem W, Mergental H, Heaton N, Mirza D, Perera MTPR, et al. Liver transplantation after ex vivo normothermic machine preservation: A phase 1 (first-in-man) clinical trial. American Journal of Transplantation. 2016;**16**(6):1779-1787

[65] Eshmuminov D, Becker D, Bautista Borrego L, Hefti M, Schuler MJ, Hagedorn C, et al. An integrated perfusion machine preserves injured human livers for 1 week. Nature Biotechnology. Feb 2020;**38**(2):189-198

[66] Boteon YL, Laing RW, Schlegel A, Wallace L, Smith A, Attard J, et al. Combined hypothermic and normothermic machine perfusion improves functional recovery of extended criteria donor livers. Liver Transplantation. 2018;**24**:1699-1715. DOI: 10.1002/lt.25315

[67] Nasralla D, Coussios CC, Mergental H, Akhtar MZ, Butler AJ, Ceresa CDL, et al. A randomized trial of normothermic preservation in liver transplantation. Nature. 2018;**557**:50-56

[68] Mergental H, Perera MT, Laing RW, Muiesan P, Isaac JR, Smith A, et al. Transplantation of declined liver allografts following normothermic ex-situ evaluation. American Journal of Transplantation. 2016;**16**:3235-3245. DOI: 10.1111/ajt.13875

[69] Matton APM, de Vries Y, Burlage LC, et al. Biliary bicarbonate, pH and glucose are suitable biomarkers of biliary viability during ex situ normothermic machine perfusion of human donor livers. Transplantation. Jul 2019;**103**(7):1405-1413

[70] Goldaracena N, Barbas AS, Selzner M. Normothermic and Subnoromothermic ex vivo liver perfusion in liver transplantation. Current Opinion in Organ Transplantation. 2016;**21**:315-321

[71] Bruinsma BG, Yeh H, Ozer S, et al. Subnormothermic machine perfusion

for ex vivo preservation and recovery of the human liver for transplantation. American Journal of Transplantation. 2014;**14**:1400-1409

[72] Minor T, Efferz P, Fox M, et al. Controlled oxygenated rewarming of cold stored liver grafts by thermally graduated machine perfusion prior to reperfusion. American Journal of Transplantation. 2013;**13**:1450-1460

[73] van Leeuwen OB, de Vries Y, Fujiyoshi M, Nijsten MWN, Ubbink R, Pelgrim GJ, et al. Transplantation of high-risk donor livers after ex situ resuscitation and assessment using combined hypo- and Normothermic machine perfusion: A prospective clinical trial. Annals of Surgery. Nov 2019;**270**(5):906-914

[74] Jamieson RW, Zilvetti M, Roy D, et al. Hepatic steatosis and normothermic perfusion-preliminary experiments in a por- cine model. Transplantation. 2011;**92**:289-295. DOI: 10.1097/TP.0b013e318223d817

[75] Nagrath D, Xu H, Tanimura Y, et al. Metabolic preconditioning of donor organs: Defatting fatty livers by normothermic perfusion ex vivo. Metabolic Engineering. 2009;**11**:274-283. DOI: 10.1016/j. ymben.2009.05.005

[76] Boteon YL, Attard J, Boteon APCS, et al. Manipulation of lipid metabolism during normothermic machine perfusion: Effect of defatting therapies on donor liver functional recovery. Liver Transplantation. 2019;**25**:1007-1022

[77] Hara Y, Akamatsu Y, Maida K, et al. A new liver graft preparation method for uncontrolled non-heart-beating donors, combining short oxygenated warm perfusion and prostaglandin E1. The Journal of Surgical Research. 2013;**184**:1134-1142. DOI: 10.1016/j.jss.2013.04.030

[78] Maida K, Akamatsu Y, Hara Y, et al. Short oxygenated warm perfusion with prostaglandin E1 administration before cold preservation as a novel resuscitation method for liver grafts from donors after car- diac death in a rat in vivo model. Transplantation. 2016;**100**:1052-1058. DOI: 10.1097/TP.0000000000001127

[79] Guarrera JV, Karim NA. Liver preservation: Is there anything new yet? Current Opinion in Organ Transplantation. 2008;**13**:148-154. DOI: 10.1097/MOT.0b013e3282f63930]

[80] Nassar A, Liu Q, Farias K, et al. Role of vasodilation during normo- thermic machine perfusion of DCD porcine livers. The International Journal of Artificial Organs. 2014;**37**:165-172. DOI: 10.5301/ijao.5000297

[81] Echeverri J, Goldaracena N, Kaths JM, et al. Comparison of BQ123, epoprostenol, and verapamil as vasodilators during normothermic ex vivo liver machine perfusion. Transplantation. 2018;**102**:601-608. DOI: 10.1097/TP.0000000000002021

[82] Goldaracena N, Spetzler VN, Echeverri J, et al. Inducing hepatitis C virus resistance after pig liver transplantation-a proof of con- cept of liver graft modification using warm ex vivo perfusion. American Journal of Transplantation. 2017;**17**:970-978. DOI: 10.1111/ajt.14100

[83] Gillooly AR, Perry J, Martins PN. First report of siRNA uptake (for RNA interference) during ex vivo hypothermic and normother- mic liver machine perfusion. Transplantation. 2019;**103**:e56-e57. DOI: 10.1097/TP.0000000000002515

[84] Thijssen MF, Brüggenwirth IMA, Gillooly A, et al. Gene silencing with siRNA (RNA interference): A new

therapeutic option during ex vivo machine liver perfusion preservation. Liver Transplantation. 2019;**25**:140-151. DOI: 10.1002/lt.25383

[85] Brüggenwirth IMA, Martins PN. RNA interference therapeutics in organ transplantation: The dawn of a new era. American Journal of Transplantation. 2020;**20**:931-941. DOI: 10.1111/ajt.15689

[86] Yu Y, Cheng Y, Pan Q, et al. Effect of the selective NLRP3 inflammasome inhibitor mcc950 on transplantation outcome in a pig liver transplantation model with organs from donors after circulatory death preserved by hypothermic machine perfusion. Transplantation. 2019;**103**:353-362. DOI: 10.1097/TP.0000000000002461

[87] Beal EW, Kim JL, Reader BF, et al. [D-Ala2, D-Leu5] Enkephalin improves liver preservation during normothermic ex vivo perfusion. The Journal of Surgical Research. 2019;**241**:323-335. DOI: 10.1016/j.jss.2019.04.010

[88] Rigo F, De Stefano N, Navarro-Tableros V, et al. Extracellular vesicles from human liver stem cells reduce injury in an ex vivo normothermic hypoxic rat liver perfusion model. Transplantation. 2018;**102**:e205-e210. DOI: 10.1097/TP.0000000000002123

[89] Jochmans I, Moers C, Smits JM, et al. Machine perfusion versus cold storage for the preservation of kidneys donated after cardiac death: A multicenter, randomized, controlled trial. Annals of Surgery. 2010;**252**:756

[90] Kron P, Schlegel A, Muller X, Gaspert A, Clavien P-A, Dutkowski P. Hypothermic oxygenated perfusion (HOPE) – A simple and effective method to modulate the immune response in kidney transplantation. Transplantation. May 2019;**103**(5):e128-e136

[91] Bellini MI, Nozdrin M, Yiu J, Papalois V. Machine perfusion for abdominal organ preservation: A systematic review of kidney and liver human grafts. Journal of Clinical Medicine. 2019;**8**(8):1221. DOI: 10.3390/jcm8081221

[92] Husen P, Boffa C, Jochmans I, Krikke C, Davies L, Mazilescu L, et al. Oxygenated end-hypothermic machine perfusion in expanded criteria donor kidney transplant: A randomized clinical trial. JAMA Surgery. 1 Jun 2021;**156**(6):517-525

[93] Jochmans I, Brat A, Davies L, Hofker HS, van de Leemkolk FEM, Leuvenink HGD, et al. Compare trial collaboration and consortium for organ preservation in Europe (COPE). Oxygenated versus standard cold perfusion preservation in kidney transplantation (COMPARE): A randomised, double-blind, paired, phase 3 trial. Lancet. 2020;**396**(10263):1653-1662

[94] Gallinat A, Amrillaeva V, Hoyer DP, Kocabayoglu P, Benko T, Treckmann JW, et al. Reconditioning by end-ischemic hypothermic in-house machine perfusion: A promising strategy to improve outcome in expanded criteria donors kidney transplantation. Clinical Transplantation. Mar 2017;**31**(3)

[95] Jochmans I, Moers C, Smits JM, Leuvenink HG, Treckmann J, Paul A, et al. The prognostic value of renal resistance during hypothermic machine perfusion of deceased donor kidneys. American Journal of Transplantation. 2011;**11**:2214-2220. DOI: 10.1111/j.1600-6143.2011.03685.x

[96] Jochmans I, Pirenne J. Graft quality assessment in kidney transplantation: Not an exact science yet! Current Opinion in Organ Transplantation.

2011;**16**:174-179. DOI: 10.1097/MOT.0b013e3283446b31

[97] Dare AJ, Pettigrew GJ, Saeb-Parsy K. Preoperative assessment of the deceased-donor kidney: From macroscopic appearance to molecular biomarkers. Transplantation. 2014;**97**:797-807. DOI: 10.1097/01.TP.0000441361.34103.53

[98] Ding CG, Li Y, Tian XH, et al. Predictive score model for delayed graft function based on hypothermic machine perfusion variables in kidney transplantation. Chinese Medical Journal. 2018;**131**:2651-2657

[99] Kox J, Moers C, Monbaliu D, Strelniece A, Treckmann J, Jochmans I, et al. The benefits of hypothermic machine preservation and short cold ischemia times in deceased donor kidneys. Transplantation. 2018;**102**:1344-1350. DOI: 10.1097/TP.0000000000002188

[100] Hosgood SA, Nicholson ML. First in man renal transplantation after ex vivo normothermic perfusion. Transplantation. 2011;**92**:735-738. DOI: 10.1097/TP.0b013e31822d4e04

[101] Nicholson ML, Hosgood SA. Renal transplantation after ex vivo normothermic perfusion: The first clinical study. American Journal of Transplantation. 2013;**13**:1246-1252. DOI: 10.1111/ajt.12179

[102] Hosgood SA, van Heurn E, Nicholson ML. Normothermic machine perfusion of the kidney: Better conditioning and repair? Transplant International. 2015;**28**:657-664

[103] Weissenbacher A, Lo Faro L, Boubriak O, et al. Twenty-four-hour normothermic perfusion of discarded human kidneys with urine recirculation. American Journal of Transplantation. 2019;**19**:178-192

[104] Hosgood SA, Barlow AD, Hunter JP, Nicholson ML. Ex vivo normothermic perfusion for quality assessment of marginal donor kidney transplants. The British Journal of Surgery. 2015;**102**:1433-1440. DOI: 10.1002/bjs.9894

[105] Gregorini M, Corradetti V, Pattonieri EF, et al. Perfusion of isolated rat kidney with mesenchymal stromal cells/extracellular vesicles prevents ischaemic injury. Journal of Cellular and Molecular Medicine. 2017;**21**:3381-3393. DOI: 10.1111/jcmm.13249

[106] Bhattacharjee RN, Richard-Mohamed M, Sun Q, et al. CORM-401 reduces ischemia reperfusion injury in an ex vivo renal porcine model of the donation after circulatory death. Transplantation. 2018;**102**:1066-1074. DOI: 10.1097/TP.0000000000002201

[107] Hamaoui K, Gowers S, Boutelle M, et al. Organ pretreatment with cytotopic endothelial localizing peptides to ameliorate microvascular thrombosis and perfusion deficits in ex vivo renal hemoreperfusion models. Transplantation. 2016;**100**:e128-e139. DOI: 10.1097/TP.0000000000001437

[108] Sedigh A, Nordling S, Carlsson F, et al. Perfusion of porcine kidneys with macromolecular heparin reduces early ischemia reperfusion injury. Transplantation. 2019;**103**:420-427. DOI: 10.1097/TP.0000000000002469

[109] Brasile L, Henry N, Orlando G, et al. Potentiating renal regeneration using mesenchymal stem cells. Transplantation. 2019;**103**:307-313. DOI: 10.1097/TP.0000000000002455

[110] Yang B, Hosgood SA, Bagul A, et al. Erythropoietin regulates apop- tosis, inflammation and tissue remodelling via caspase-3 and IL-1β in isolated hemoperfused kidneys. European Journal

of Pharmacology. 2011;**660**:420-430. DOI: 10.1016/j.ejphar.2011.03.044

[111] Yang C, Hosgood SA, Meeta P, et al. Cyclic helix B peptide in preservation solution and autologous blood perfusate ameliorates ischemia-reperfusion injury in isolated porcine kidneys. Transplantation direct. 2015;**1**:e6. DOI: 10.1097/TXD.0000000000000515

[112] Zhang Y, Wang Q, Liu A, Wu Y, Liu F, Wang H, et al. Erythropoietin derived peptide improved endoplasmic reticulum stress and ischemia-reperfusion related cellular and renal injury. Frontiers in Medicine (Lausanne). 2020;7:5. DOI: 10.3389/fmed.2020.00005

[113] Tietjen GT, Hosgood SA, DiRito J, et al. Nanoparticle targeting to the endothelium during normothermic machine perfusion of human kidneys. Science Translational Medicine. 2017;**9**:eaam6764. DOI: 10.1126/scitranslmed.aam6764

[114] Giwa S, Lewis JK, Alvarez L, et al. The promise of organ and tissue preservation to transform medicine. Nature Biotechnology. 2017;**35**(6): 530-542

[115] Schlegel A, Muller X, Dutkowski P. Machine perfusion strategies in liver transplantation. Hepatobiliary Surgery and Nutrition. 2019;**8**(5):490-501. DOI: 10.21037/hbsn.2019.04.04